HITCH FIT

KEYS TO

TRANSFORMING

YOUR LIFE

MICAH LACERTE

&

DIANA CHALOUX

NOTES OF GRATITUDE
FROM MICAH

I want to say thank you to those people who have stuck by my side through thick and thin during this journey - the ones who always believed in me when it seemed my dreams were bigger than possibly attainable. You are a main reason I'm here today doing what I'm doing. Through the years I have let many people go and also met people who will remain in my life forever. This I believe is what helps us grow and teaches us what life is about. Your positive comfort and lending ear have kept my goals and dreams within grasp.

First off, I want to say thank you to my mother, father, grandparents and uncles. You have been my foundation and were always my biggest supporters and fans. Diana, I love you with all my heart. You have helped me to grow and understand what true love is all about. I feel so blessed to be able to spend the rest of my life with you!

Next are my best friends. You have always been there for me in times of hardship and times I wanted to give up. Thank you for your consistent support and love. I am truly blessed to have you in my life.

I want to thank my amazing clients whom I have been able to work with over the years. Through your transformations, I myself have transformed. Through you, I have found my true passion in life: helping others. To all the rest of you who were there for a reason or a season, thank you for your guidance and support.

In my life I have learned some very valuable lessons; some by making bad choices and some through people who shared their life with me. When times are tough, stay positive and surround yourself with people who will help you to be the best you can be. I am truly thankful and blessed to have all these people in my life.

I love you and I'm always here for you.   -Micah LaCerte

NOTES OF GRATITUDE
FROM DIANA

I have to start by saying how grateful I am to God for giving such a wonderful, unique and positive opportunity to Micah and I. Working in the fitness industry and having the ability to aid others in leading more healthy and fit lifestyles is such an amazing way to spend this life. I couldn't ask for anything better.

I want to say thank you to my amazing family. Without their unconditional love and support I don't believe I would be where I'm at today. I was never discouraged from chasing my dreams, and even though I've screwed up a lot of things in my life, I never doubted for a second that they would be there to pick me up and dust me off.

Thank you to my father Frank and his wife Dorothy, and my mother Rosie and her husband Mark. Thank you to my beautiful sister Maria. A special thank you to my big sister Linda who has been the wind beneath my wings, my best friend and my right hand woman since my journey in fitness began. She supported me and put a roof over my head, and I literally would not have achieved half of the dreams and goals that were placed in my heart. To my brother in law Scott, thank you for being so amazingly tolerant and gracious.

I'd of course like to say thank you to Micah. From the first time that we met I knew that my life would never be the same. You are the one person that I never knew I needed, and now I can't imagine living without. I love you with all my heart, I'm so grateful that we are partners in all things. I love my life with you, and I can't wait to continue on this journey that God has set out for us.

To my dear friends and clients, I feel so blessed to have had each and every one of you in my life. For those who I've had the chance to aid in becoming more fit and healthy, I am so honored to have been a part of your journey! – Love, Diana Chaloux.

CONTENTS

Motivation   i

Introduction   1

1   You Can Get There From Here   Pg 6

2   The Accident   Pg 10

3   My Moment of Re-Inspiration   Pg 13

4   Small Town Girl with a Dream   Pg 17

5   My Aha Moment   Pg 21

6   From Fat to Hitch Fit   Pg 33

7   Your Transformation = Inspiration + Perspiration   Pg 39

8   Lifestyle: Keys to Happiness   Pg 44

9   Motivation + Transformation   Pg 65

10   Nutrition   Pg 82

11   Fitness   Pg 110

12   Final Thoughts   Pg 131

MOTIVATION

Our main goal in life is to listen to God and go where He asks us to go, to love and to laugh, to wake up every day happy, and to aid as many people as possible in living a healthier, happier and more fit lifestyle.

Thanks for reading this book. We hope that it inspires you even a little bit, and always know that if there's any way that we, Micah and Diana, can help you, we are happy to do so!

INTRODUCTION

We would first like to say thank you so much for taking the time to read this book. We know that there are so many different ways you can spend your valuable time, and to have you choose to use it allowing us to share a bit of our journey and some knowledge means a lot to us!

What is Hitch Fit?

Hitch Fit is a lifestyle. It's about changing your mind, your body and ultimately your life and fulfilling your true potential throughout your journey here on earth.

Hitch Fit was the original concept of Micah "Hitch" LaCerte. Micah is one of the nation's top personal trainers, a professional fitness model with multiple features and covers in magazines such as Muscle & Fitness, Status Fitness, Maximum Fitness, Men's Workout, Exercise for Men, and WBFF Fit and Firm. Micah is a WBFF Pro athlete, actor, motivational speaker, author and columnist for Status Fitness Magazine as well as a coach. Micah discovered from an early age that his passion was within the fitness industry, and once he experienced the joy of aiding his first clients in physical transformation, he became hooked on the experience of having such a positive, long lasting impact on someone else's life. In 2008, Micah met Diana Chaloux, and as soon as these two met, sparks flew in more ways than one.

Shortly after meeting, Micah and Diana recognized that their life passions were both the same, and that there was a spark between them that neither had experienced before. Diana is an ACE Certified Personal Trainer and graduated at the top of her class at Fitness Professionals International. She is also a successful fitness model and

WBFF Pro athlete, having claimed multiple top placements in the world of competition including two World Champion titles. She is a Well coach certified fitness coach and AFPA certified nutritionist. She has been featured in multiple nationwide publications including Oxygen Women's Fitness, Status Fitness, Muscle and Fitness Hers, Natural Muscle, World Physique and MMA Worldwide.

Within two months of meeting at the Olympia Weekend in Las Vegas, Diana had packed up her life in San Antonio, Texas and moved up to Kansas City to be with Micah. Quick decision? Yes, but Diana had absolutely no doubts or hesitancy, knowing that she had met the man of her dreams.

Micah and Diana pooled their knowledge and ideas together to do the official launch of Hitch Fit online training in February 2009. A few short months later in July 2009, the two had the opportunity to open their own personal training studio in Kansas City, and jumped at the chance to have a physical location to continue to grow the company and change lives.

Hitch Fit is about so much more than just personal training. It is about transformation: true mind, body and spirit transformation. It's not about trying to get clients in for training and then trying to retain them for long periods of time. The goal is to provide our clients, whether online or in person, with the tools that they need to transform their bodies and their lifestyles in order to ultimately be healthier, happier and to lead a higher quality -- and in many cases -- quantity of life.

Micah and Diana were blessed to have people around them who believed in them, and saw the potential for what Hitch Fit could grow to become. With that support system in place, Hitch Fit experienced amazing growth in its first year! When Micah and Diana united, there was no turning back! The now notorious, Hitch Fit "Wall of Transformations" more than tripled in size within an 8-month period of time as people began to see their friends or family members undergoing remarkable inside/out transformations.

Micah and Diana are committed to seeing Hitch Fit grow and thrive in an effort to bring the good word of healthy living to people of all walks of life, young and old, male or female, obese or those who are in decent shape looking to be in "rock star" shape.

Welcome to Hitch Fit

Welcome to the world of Hitch Fit. If you are just beginning your fitness journey we encourage you to dream big, to never doubt your true potential, and to dig deep down inside yourself and find the courage, the strength and the determination to reach a higher level of success and happiness in your life. All of which you have potential for and deserve. We are grateful to be a part of this adventure with you!

Our goal with each person we work with, whether online or in person, is to encourage them to take a deeper look inside themselves, to earn their trust and teach them not only how to become fit and healthy, but ultimately to be happier and more fulfilled with their lives. If we can inspire even one person to make positive changes in their life then we will have succeeded.

Our personal motivation for doing what we do, for writing this book, and for working in this industry, come from different places. But the main drive comes from knowing without a shadow of a doubt that God has placed this passion to help others deep in our hearts and souls, and this is 100% the path that He has laid out for us.

What's your story?

Each person has a different story, experiences that have shaped them, life experiences peppered with struggles and trials which only serve to make you stronger and better as a person. We will both share our personal stories with you in this book so that you will know a bit of the struggles we have been through as well. But as you begin reading this book, it's now time to start asking yourself some deep and important questions. What type of person are you?

As we tell our stories, we want you to think about your own. We all have one; we all have had different experiences and made choices that have brought us to the place we are at today. What has happened to you in this life that has held you back, either emotionally or physically, in making the best healthy choices for yourself? Perhaps you have struggled with being overweight or obese your entire life, or maybe like Micah you struggled with the opposite, being a hard gainer and being teased because you were "skinny". Are you someone who expresses your emotions openly or do you hold everything in, and avoid showing your true feelings? You may have struggled in the past with abuse, with insecurity, with broken relationships, divorce, death, illness or injury. Or perhaps as you grew older, life just took over in the form of busy jobs and busy family life, and in the midst of it all, you forgot to take care of you. Maybe it's not any of those scenarios... perhaps you are in a great place in your life, making great choices, and are ready to take your fitness to the next level via a fitness competition. Regardless of where you are in your life, what your goals are, what your past obstacles are, or what choices you've made, we are happy to have you as part of our team.

Regardless of where you are right now -- physically, emotionally, mentally and spiritually -- we will share with you ways that you can eliminate any negatives and get your life focused in the most positive direction! Please be prepared to do some soul searching and be completely honest with yourself about how you have dealt with your past hurts and trials, and be prepared to let go of old excuses and obstacles in order to take full grasp of what you can truly achieve!

Follow us through this process, make positive choices and be willing to make the necessary sacrifices that it will take to get to where you want to be. You must TAKE THE RISK. If you don't, you will never know what your true potential could have been. Failure is not an option. Your focus must be on your ability to succeed!

Transformation is never easy. There's no sugar coating or empty promises here. It will take hard work, determination, discipline and sacrifice. But through this, you WILL find yourself and become the person you have always known was there. Never give up, work hard, stay focused and know inside that you have the ability to become a better you.

CHAPTER 1
YOU CAN GET THERE FROM HERE
Micah's Story: Part 1

People ask me on a regular basis, "How did you get where you are today, and how can I get there?"

I started my personal transformation at the age of 19. I had just started college and was unhappy with what I looked like. I was an athlete growing up, but I was called skinny and taunted with names like "chicken legs"- one that one always stuck in my mind. I was 6 feet, 150 pounds when I graduated from high school. I was always a "hard gainer," which is fitness lingo for someone who has a difficult time gaining weight no matter how much they eat or how hard they work out.

I couldn't gain a pound. Patience was always my enemy. I wanted instant gratification. I wanted everything to happen NOW. I soon realized that this was not going to happen. As with all good things in life, this was going to take hard work and dedication. It wasn't going to happen overnight. I started reading fitness magazines and books, watched fitness- and wellness-based television shows. I wanted the perfect body. That was my goal. That was my motivation.

Over time, I had become insecure with my appearance. To make things worse, on the outside I would act as though everything was fine, but I held a lot of pain on the inside for years. I had endured experiences in my childhood and adolescence that no human being should ever have to endure.

I no longer wanted to feel insecure about being skinny. I made a choice that would change my life forever. My choice was to eliminate everything from my life that would prevent me from achieving a perfect physique. This included ending negative relationships, structuring my lifestyle in a way that was conducive to achieving my fitness goals, ending partying, drinking and other activities that would only hold me back from success.

After of few years of figuring out my workouts, my lifestyle and my nutrition, I achieved - in my mind - what I had set out to do. By the age of 23, I had gained nearly 30 pounds and reduced my body fat to 2 to 4%. Interestingly enough, though, I realized that through this whole process, my goals had changed.

I had transformed myself and found that by doing so, I now had a deep desire to show others how they could do the same. I had developed a passion for the fitness industry and started personal training in college. I earned my degree in business marketing, but at that point I wasn't concerned about finding a high-paying job in that field.

I knew I was only going to be happy if I followed my passion and continued down the fitness track. I knew that pursuing a different career just because of how much money I could earn was a dead-end road if I wanted to be content and happy in my life. Money comes and goes and is not the key to happiness. I realized that to be as successful as possible in the fitness industry, I had to be a walking billboard of fitness and wellness.

So that's literally what I did. I wanted everything that I was preaching to be exactly how I was living. I started focusing on making the right choices in every aspect of my life and becoming over-all HAPPY. I refused to be that trainer in the gym that was overweight and out of shape while preaching to clients about eating right, living right and working out. I wanted my clients and people in my life to respect the fact that I put so much effort and passion into what I do not only for myself but because I care about their well-being and want to be a positive role model for them.

After a few years of personal training, I knew I was going to stay in this field for the rest of my life. I felt the desire to push myself even farther. I knew that I had a great story to tell that could provide inspiration to a lot of people. I had overcome a lot of adversity in my life and come out a positive healthy and happy individual. I knew that millions of people around the world would be able to relate to my experiences and that my story could help them overcome the challenges in their own lives.

My next challenge was finding a way to reach these people. How was I going to reach a worldwide audience? My path of choice was the world of fitness modeling. Achieving success within the fitness industry was the perfect opportunity to build a name and reputation that would give me a platform to speak from and share with people the secrets of living positive, fit, healthy and happy.

I focused on being published in nationwide magazines, seen on national television - anything and everything that would give me the opportunity to get my name out there so I could share my story. Throughout the process, I encountered many skeptics, including friends and girlfriends who said I would never make it. Since I knew that to be the best I could be I had to cut every aspect of negativity out of my life, I had to remove these people from my life.

I kept the people who loved me and believed in me very close. They were the support that I needed through this hard process. I stayed focused on a dream that I knew one day would be my reality. I spent more than four years working tirelessly to get my portfolio the best it could be. My entire focus was on achieving my dream. I invested every dime that I had in order to develop the essential elements for this career path.

I invested in photo shoots, traveling expenses, marketing and ultimately developing the best portfolio and resume that I could. I networked with people and continually built up my contact list in order to get in front of the right people who would ultimately aid me in achieving my dream. I stayed in top shape year round just in case I ever got the call to do a photo shoot.

My biggest obstacle was location. Most of the top male fitness models were living in Los Angeles, Miami and New York. I was living in Kansas City, which is a great place, but not for the type of modeling I was doing. I wanted this to be home base in order to be close to my family. I made frequent trips to LA, Miami and NY, all the spots that would get me the exposure I needed. I marketed myself to everyone I met, a necessity in this highly competitive industry.

My hard work resulted in being published in more than 30 national magazines, I was featured on two nationwide magazine covers, three television reality shows, more than 50 commercials and even served as a judge for the Miss USA and Miss America pageants. Despite the success that I was achieving, I realized that it was very important to stay humble and grounded because ultimately my underlying motivation is to help others. Little did I know that everything could change in the blink of an eye.

CHAPTER 2
THE ACCIDENT
Micah's Story: Part 2

I was at the peak of my career in the summer of 2005. I was at the top of my game, one of the top male fitness models in the country. I had recently been featured on the reality show "Manhunt," landed the cover of Men's Workout magazine and had features in multiple other publications. Everything was going in the right direction toward my dreams and goals. I was at a crossroads, trying to make major career choices.

My options were wide open. With all of the nationwide exposure, things were certainly overwhelming, but I was at the happiest point in my life, on top of the world. I could move to LA and pursue modeling and a role on a popular soap opera show or I could stay in Kansas City and pursue the projects that I had been building on there. Little did I know that in one split second, my life was about to change completely…that everything I had worked so hard to achieve was going to be snatched away from me in a heartbeat.

The car accident that rocked my world and completely altered my destiny happened in June 2005. I was driving to the airport with my mother and a friend, on my way to Florida for a job.

As we were driving down the highway at 65 miles per hour, a ladder fell off the vehicle in front of us and landed in the middle of the road. We were in a small vehicle and attempted to swerve out of the way of the ladder in order to avoid flipping the car. There was a truck to our right, which we hit, and then our car was pummeled by another vehicle.

It was a messy accident, and I knew right off the bat I was in trouble.

The force of the impact caused major whiplash and a hip injury resulting in severe back and neck issues for me. My livelihood at that point in my life was fitness and working out, not only keeping myself in tip-top condition but also aiding others in achieving their fitness goals and staying motivated.

Initially I tried to fight through the pain and continue on with my life as it had been before, but it became too much. I needed chiropractic work 3 to 5 days a week and would have to continue that process for more than six months. In addition it was going to take 6- to 9- months of treatment to get my hips re-aligned. The doctors told me that I could not work out, but I couldn't endure the pain of it anyway.

The physical achievements I had attained started to deteriorate before my eyes. I fell into a state of depression and was unmotivated. I lost my mojo. I lost my strength, flexibility and 30- pounds of my hard-earned muscle. I became withdrawn from the passions that made me happy. I lost my look as a fitness model and didn't have the size that I needed to be working in that portion of the industry any longer.

On top of that, I wasn't able to work as much anymore to pay my bills and to get myself out to LA or NY to do the shoots in the first place. I was frustrated, depressed and waking up in the morning completely unhappy. Every time I looked in the mirror, I helplessly watched my body go from magazine cover shape back to what I had started with when I was 18 years old.

My life began to go on a downward spiral. I started living a different lifestyle. I had lost hope in myself and accepted that I would never be able to achieve the goals I had set. I felt like I was an utter disappointment to the people who had believed in me. At that point it seemed that all my hard work was wasted.

I started living for unsatisfying momentary pleasures instead of doing things that would allow me to pursue and achieve my goals. I was living paycheck to paycheck, just trying to stay afloat. I started making extremely poor lifestyle choices. I was staying out late, partying and drinking, eating whatever I wanted. Go to a typical club - I was that guy, out there on Thursday, Friday and Saturday night, living it up, hanging out with the wrong crowd in the wrong environment.

I had preached healthy living and kept positive people and surroundings around me for so long, then suddenly I found myself in this completely negative environment. If you knew me before, you would realize that just wasn't me. If I were to go out before, I was drinking water or I may have had one drink and call it good. During this phase of my life I was getting tipsy if not drunk on a regular basis. I wasn't used to this lifestyle.

This wasn't the definition of who I was. I had gone from being completely motivated and passionate, a rock star, to simply not caring about anything. I was trying to pillow the feelings I had inside by living a lifestyle that had never been suitable for my goals or me.

Then, as quickly as my hope had been taken away, it was given back.

CHAPTER 3
MY MOMENT OF RE-INSPIRATION
Micah's story: Part 3

It was late November 2007 when I got the call from a friend in LA that became a turning point for me. While she was browsing through the magazines in a nutritional store, she noticed I was on the cover of the latest edition of Muscle and Body magazine. When she called to tell me, I was in a state of disbelief. I said, "What? I haven't shot anything in over a year! Where is this coming from?"

As it turns out the cover shot was a picture of me with top female fitness model Jennifer Nicole Lee. It was the January 2007 cover, but this was a photo shoot that we had done over two years ago in 2005. There had been a lapse of a year, to a year and a half, since I had even done any shoots at this point in time. Needless to say, I was excited. This was the motivation I needed to reach my goals.

Seeing myself on that cover sparked my desire and my will to succeed once again. I had forgotten about the person that I once was, but now that my memory had been refreshed, I wanted to be him again. The change in me was almost instant. I woke up the next morning, looked at myself in the mirror and said, "Today is the day that I change in every single way."

I decided to give my dreams another shot by putting 100% effort towards achieving the goals I had set over 2 years before. I knew how much work and sacrifice it was going to take, but it was a challenge I needed-and wanted. The first thing I did was sit down and reassess my entire life situation. What did I need to do to get back to the point I had been at prior to my accident?

I sat down and wrote out a list of goals. I also made a list of all the negative factors that were in my life, including the people and places that should no longer be a part of my life. Next, I made a list of the things that needed to be done in order to get back on a positive track, keep me moving toward a successful future and ultimately allow me to be happy again.

When I was able to lift again, I started back slowly. I had a lot of frustrating moments, as I had not only lost weight, I had lost the majority of my strength as well. My lack of ability to perform the way I used to in the gym made me want to scream. I struggled through days where I doubted myself, where my dreams still seemed so far away, where I questioned whether I would ever reach that elite level of fitness again.

It was on these days that I had to dig down even deeper in order to find the motivation to continue pressing forward. When I did that, I discovered that I possessed an inner strength and the ability to overcome all of my obstacles, and over time, I found I could not only be the person I once was, I could actually become an even better version of my former self. I was happier and healthier in all aspects of my life.

I refused to feel sorry for myself any longer. I started working out hard, got my diet back on track, got back to sprinting on the track and basically revamped my entire lifestyle. I surrounded myself once again with positive people and places and within a short period of time I was on my way to being in my best condition ever. Even better, I was getting Micah back.

I shared my challenges with others when the story I am telling you now was published in a nationwide fitness magazine. Through all of this I had been given just the opportunity I wanted, to share my story with a huge audience and offer them hope and inspiration to overcome their own personal obstacles in order to achieve health and happiness.

You have the chance to show people that regardless of the negatives that you have experienced in your life; you have the choice to turn them into something positive.

It may take a year or five years, but through it you have to keep that drive, will and strength as strong as possible to get to the place in your life where you ultimately want to be.

Today my fundamental drive, my underlying motivation doesn't come from working out or trying to attain physical perfection. It comes from the desire to help people.

I get so much fulfillment and happiness out of teaching people and talking to people about how to make the right choices in their life. That is where the life-coaching portion of this program comes into play. Though I didn't realize it at the time, I can see clearly now that every trial and struggle I had to go through in order to reach this place has been worth it.

These challenges were blessings in disguise. They opened my eyes to the fact that anything can happen at any point in your life. You may have to work through struggle but you CAN come out on top. We've all made choices in our lives that weren't the best ones.

You may believe that you have no way out due to a controllable or uncontrollable situation. But there is a way out. There are always choices to be made. You have to reach a level where you literally say, "Enough is enough."

You have to have the desire to get to a different level, to be happy, to be successful and to find that underlying motivation that will drive you to a better place and finally allow you to be a positive, healthy and happy individual.

The last few years, I have dedicated my life to teaching people how to become successful through positive choices and healthy living. I live and teach by the motto, "Live healthy. Live happy." If you become happy with who you are, you will be able to make others happy. I have never smiled more in my life than I have recently.

The more success I achieve personally, the more I am able to aid others in achieving their own success. I am grateful to live such a blessed and purposeful life. I'm living proof that you can and WILL reach your goals regardless of the struggles you have been through. I hope to provide you with inspiration and am honored to be a part of your journey to a more positive, successful, fit and healthy, happy place in life. Now it's time for you to make the choice. Are you ready? You are worth it!

CHAPTER FOUR
SMALL TOWN GIRL WITH A DREAM
Diana's Story: Part 1

My story is quite different than Micah's. Somehow we both had completely different paths in life that eventually coincided at just the right time for us to come together and create Hitch Fit.

My love affair with physical fitness started at an early age. I grew up in the beautiful little state of Vermont, in a small town called St. Johnsbury. I loved sports, though I was far from being a star athlete in any sense of the word. From a young age, my parents had me participating in basketball, cross country running, gymnastics and swimming.

I was never the biggest, the best, the fastest, the strongest, or the most graceful (I'm sure my gymnastics coaches would strongly agree with that!). I was clumsy (still am!!) and a little pudgy when I was a kid, my sisters even gave me the delightful nickname "Diana Cabana the Big Fat Banana", (though they were scolded profusely by mom and dad if caught calling me that)! But not having the highest skill level never stopped me from absolutely loving sports, from working as hard as I could and giving my whole heart to whatever it was I was attempting to achieve.

Actually, I believe that not being naturally gifted at sports caused me to work even harder than I would have otherwise, knowing that the only way I was going to make the basketball team was if I improved on my left-handed layups, causing me to relentlessly practice until I got better. The other driving force for me was the fact that my little sister Maria was a very natural athlete. I never wanted my little sister to beat me, so I worked my tail off twice as hard to make sure I could stay a couple steps ahead of her. She kept me on my toes for sure.

I was first introduced to the weight room at age 14. I was dating a guy who was on the high school football team, and he would get up early in the mornings and get to school an hour early in order to work out. He invited me to come along, and I thought it sounded like fun.

Honestly, at that point in my life, with no outside guidance and having never even read a fitness magazine, I had NO clue what I was doing. I would mimic what I saw other people doing, and ended up doing loads of leg press, bench press, leg extensions and the abs crunch machine. I didn't know exactly what muscle groups I was working (though now looking back I definitely attribute the development of my quads to all those leg presses and extensions, and the mass of my upper abdominals can be traced back to that crazy old abs machine), but I knew that it felt good. I loved how I felt after workouts. I loved how strong I felt and how confident.

I was painfully shy (not kidding…PAINFULLY…to the point where I would almost have a panic attack if asked to speak in class) when I began high school. The gym and sports were what helped me come out of my shell and gain confidence in myself and the young woman I was becoming. I still didn't know exactly what I wanted to become, but I remember wanting so badly to be a Pro at something, to be the best at something, to be number one at something.

Strength training remained a fairly consistent part of my life over the course of the next 7 years. I played basketball in college and worked out on a regular basis. But despite that, college was also the first time in my life that I started to struggle with my weight. Some gain the freshman 15, I gained the freshman 30. It was all due to my own poor choices! College life granted me a freedom that I had never known before, and I will be the first to admit that I was a bit of a party animal!

The consequences of those choices snuck up on me quicker than I imagined, and I found myself majorly struggling with body image issues. I was mad at myself for letting this happen to me, yet at the same time, I wasn't willing yet to make different choices for myself.

Entering my sophomore year, the initial allure of college living had worn off slightly. I won't lie and say that I stopped being a little party girl, but I realized that as I was getting older I couldn't get away with just eating whatever I wanted anymore. I did lose some of that initial weight gain as I cut back on some of the junk I was eating, and started running on a regular basis. Unfortunately, I still had no good direction or guidance in this area, I was subject to the mass media as my main source of information when it came to health and fitness (as are most people!).

The majority of what I learned came from television (this was years before I would actually have a computer of my own). I believed that weight loss was easy, because that's what the people on the infomercials said. I thought that all I had to do to lose weight was follow one of the fad starvation diets. I also still believed that there was some type of magical abs exercise that I could do that would reveal my abdominal muscles if I did it often enough (thus my slight obsession with doing 8 minute abs videos every single day).

With these pre-conceived notions, I would literally get up in the morning, not eat breakfast, starve myself for as long as possible (which usually ended up being around 2-3 p.m.), and then I would binge. I would be so ridiculously hungry to the point where I couldn't think straight and I would go on a tirade, eating everything and anything in site. As soon as I was stuffed I would determine that I would not eat again for the rest of the day. But once evening came around, that plan was always foiled as I once again got so hungry I couldn't stand it!

I wasn't what would be considered overweight by any means during those years, but I remember how much of a mystery my body was to me. I wanted it to change, but I truly had no idea how to do it. I also was one of the firm believers that nutrition was not that big a factor and I could eat whatever I wanted as long as I was going out for runs and going to the gym. I really and truly believed that!

Throughout college, I was still trying to figure out what I wanted to do with my life. I changed majors 5 times because I was so indecisive and nothing seemed to really capture and hold my interest. I always had big dreams and big thoughts. I wanted to travel, I wanted to get away, and I wanted to BE somebody. I wanted to be special and stand out from the crowd. I just had no idea what that was, and I had no idea how a small town girl who had barely been out of Vermont was ever going to achieve those dreams and make something of herself..

CHAPTER FIVE
MY AHA MOMENT: THE PRICE IS RIGHT!
Diana's Story: Part 2

I'm a big believer that "aha" moments are catalysts that can lead to change, whether that is a change in a belief system you have about yourself, or a change in behaviors and actions. My definition of an "aha" moment is:

> *That moment when something happens, or someone says something, that sets off a light bulb in your head, switches your gears from making excuses (or being in a state of non-belief in yourself), to coming up with solutions and being ready to take action towards a goal...or simply believing in your ability to achieve the life that you want to lead.*

They can come at any time, they can be in the form of something major that happens in your life, or they can be as small as reading a quote that hits home, or someone making a comment that strikes a chord and spurs you to take action.

"Aha" moments can occur at anytime. They are crucial moments that shape the beliefs you have about yourself, and we all know that what you believe to be true of yourself is often the shape of your reality. If you tell yourself various excuses like you don't have time to lose weight, you are too busy, you can't do it because you are destined to be overweight, or even that your love for food is too strong to overcome, then those thoughts and beliefs are going to be your truth, your reality.

"Aha" moments change those beliefs and perceptions, allowing you to change your mind, which can lead to changing your choices, and ultimately can lead to changing your body and your life.

How do you know if you've had an "aha" moment? One sign is a change in thinking…a switch from the "I can't" to the "I can". You may start to see a situation, which in the past seemed overwhelming or daunting, but now you view it through new eyes and feel excitement over tackling the challenge instead of dread.

An "aha" moment sparks a feeling of empowerment, and I think creates a sense that a weight has been lifted off your shoulders. It's a release of fear, and it ignites the desire to find solutions. It does not mean that you will have an easy journey to achieve success, but it does give you the motivation to start your journey in the right direction.

I'd like to share with you a fun story, one of the most fun stories I have to share actually. I don't have a story of a tragic accident like Micah, just the reverse, one of my major "ah-ha" moments stems from an amusing experience, and something that many people dream of and hope will happen to them. This particular story has nothing to do with weight loss, but rather a moment in life that changed my thinking patterns. It's the moment in my life that my eyes were opened to the fact that it didn't matter how small a town I was from, or how daunting a goal may seem. I realized that anything, absolutely anything was possible in my life. It was the moment that I saw myself differently, I saw myself as special and capable, and it caused me to start dreaming - not just small dreams, but huge ones. Where did this moment occur for me? Believe it or not, it was on the stage at one of the most popular game shows on television, "The Price is Right".

I always knew there was a great big world out there, but going far away just seemed so out of reach for me. My junior year of college, one of my best friends invited me to come with her and her sorority sisters to California for spring break. To a small town Vermonter, that seemed like a million miles and worlds away. I decided that whatever it took, I had to somehow make this happen. I was so anxious for this trip and for what lay ahead. I was actually going through a real rough patch at that point. My parents had recently split up, and I had just gone through a nasty break-up with a college boyfriend. My circle of friends at that point consisted of the basketball teams, and since it was cooler to be on "his side" than mine, that is what the majority of my former friends chose to do.

I was sad and a bit lonely, and was actually seriously considering leaving school and joining the Air Force (following in my big sister Linda's footsteps). I had gone in and spoken with a recruiting officer and everything, I was ready to run away at that point. Something inside of me told me that wasn't right for me, but I was trying to muffle that voice as much as possible.

Most days it took all the courage I could muster to keep my head held high and go through the motions of attending classes, basketball practices and the worst time of all, going to the dining hall for lunch. I stuck my nose up in the air, pretended that the verbal attacks didn't hurt me one bit, and anxiously anticipated my upcoming journey.

The week of the trip finally came. I drove the four hours to New York in my little red Plymouth Horizon. This was the first car that I had bought completely on my own. I paid $800 for it, and my Dad made sure I had the best, studded tires for the snow he could find. Actually, the tires my Dad put on for me probably cost more than the car itself. This little beetle had carted my butt around for a good year or so. The funniest thing about this car was the fact that it didn't have a working heater. Need I remind you I lived in VERMONT, the land of freezing cold winter weather.

Driving to campus on a chilly winter morning was always a challenge! First I had to dig the little beast out of whatever snow had fallen, then desperately try to scrape all the ice off the windshield while bundled up in 3 or 4 layers of coats and sweaters, two pairs of gloves, a neck warmer and the warmest hat I could find, since there was no chance of the car heating up - no matter how long I had it running! My trip to New York was a very chilly one. I remember when I finally arrived, my lips were blue with the cold. I remember sitting on the floor at my girlfriends sorority house bundled up in a blanket for at least an hour trying to warm up my chilled bones.

The next day we flew out to California, the land of sunshine, the land of movie stars. I had such an anxious feeling about this trip. Anxious in a good way! I felt like this trip was going to somehow change my life, but I wasn't quite sure how or why.

One of the things that we had decided to do was go on "The Price is Right" while we were there. We were staying at one of the sorority sisters' homes in San Diego, but had decided to make the drive up to Hollywood and try to make it on the popular game show.

The first day we attempted to get on the show, we arrived at 5 a.m. to start our long wait in line. We didn't know that you needed to have tickets for the show in order to have a shot at getting in. They actually give out more tickets than people who can actually fit into the studio, and then it's a first-come, first-serve basis as to who actually gets in for the taping. We had to get standby tickets that day, and the only way that we would make it in was if not enough people with regular tickets showed up. That, of course, didn't happen.

There were plenty of people there with regular tickets, and after waiting for a good seven hours or so, we were sadly disappointed that we weren't going to make it in. My heart dropped. I had been so excited. The thought of being on national television was one that I couldn't quite wrap my head around. It just seemed so far out of the norm for me. I had actually told friends back home that I was going on "The Price is Right" and that I was going to win a car, so the thought of having to tell them that we didn't even make it in to the studio was crushing.

We were all upset by the turn of events, and we all agreed that we really wanted to try again the next day. This time, we got our tickets ahead of time so that we would have a shot at getting in to the studio audience. We found a cheap hotel on Santa Monica Boulevard, and seven girls crammed into one small room. I slept on the floor that night snuggled up in some shady looking hotel blankets, but I didn't really care. The fact that we had decided to be spontaneous and stay overnight to press our luck again the following day was exhilarating.

It was like déjà vu as we woke up early the following morning and groggily made our way back to CBS studios, and the line already forming for the Price is Right tapings. We were confident that we were going to make it this time around as we got there early enough to be in one of the front rows. The taping wasn't until about 1:30 p.m. so we had a lot of time to kill.

We were informed that we were all going to receive numbers, and in small groups, had an opportunity to do a brief interview with the producer of the show that day. That is how they decide who will be chosen to "Come on down".

I knew that since we had a good size group of girls, there was a chance that one of us would make it on stage. I started developing a mini speech to say to the producer when my chance arrived, hoping to capture his attention and be one of the select few.

Our big moment finally came. There were about 12 people in our group, all standing in a semi circle in front of the producer. A girl with a list of what I'm assuming were names and numbers sat huddled in the corner waiting for whatever signal it was from him as to who he had chosen.

All of the other girls in my group gave their speeches first. A couple of the girls were nervous and giggly…to be expected of course…but I felt cool as a cucumber since I had been reciting my little speech in my mind for at least three hours and knew exactly what I was going to say.

When the producer finally looked my way and said, "Tell me something about yourself". I took a deep breath and said, "Hi, my name is Diana Chaloux and I'm here today with all these crazy girls (smiled and nodded towards my exuberant flock of friends). I go to Lyndon State College in Vermont and I'm the captain of the women's basketball team there. We are all here today to give Barker's Beauties a run for their money." At that point, I cracked a huge grin at the producer, all my girlfriends erupted into "woohoo's", and the producer nodded his head and gave a little chuckle. Our group was hustled through to the studio (much smaller than I expected it to be), found our seats, and then anxiously waited for the rest of the studio to fill up and the show to begin.

As we were sitting there, the girls kept saying, "They're going to pick you!" I didn't want to get my hopes up too high, but to be totally honest, I knew that they were right. I could feel it. I just knew that it was going to happen. I felt excited, but calm, and started planning out in my head what I was going to do when they called out my name. When the show started, it moved so fast that our heads were spinning! I was anxiously waiting to hear my name, but when it didn't happen the first half of the show, my heart started to sink.

During one of the commercial break times, Bob Barker chatted with the audience and talked to our group. The girls all told him that they were from New York and that we were on spring break. The second round of the show started and I still wasn't called. At that point, I was really starting to feel sick to my stomach. Maybe I had been wrong, maybe I wasn't going to be chosen. I knew that there were only two opportunities left to be called down. Then suddenly, in an instant, I saw a giant flashcard being held up down at the front with a name on it...there it was "Diana Chaloux". There was no mistake. As I heard Rod Roddy completely slaughter my last name as he said "The next name on my list is Diana Chaloux (pronounced Sha – Lou, but he said Chal – Low), I'm not sure where she's from but she's going to come on down!" I calmly stood up and trotted to the front. I didn't jump or scream or freak out, I don't even think I turned to the girls when he called me. It's so funny because I was just expecting it to happen, so it wasn't a great surprise when it did.

Bob bantered with me a bit when I took my place on contestant's row and explained to him that I wasn't from NY, but from Vermont and that I was just here with my friends for the show. The next item

27

up for bid was a bracelet. Now mind you, at this point in my life, I didn't even know how to apply mascara, and my main "jewelry" was a hair tie that I constantly kept around my wrist in case I needed to pull my hair back into a ponytail. I had no clue what to bid on the bracelet and nervously looked back at my girlfriends for advice. I think I bid $900.00 (could be wrong, you'll have to watch the video which I have posted on my YouTube page at www.youtube.com/user/shoobydoo52) . I didn't win. I was bummed because I knew the show was coming to a close and there was only going to be one more opportunity to place a bid.

The boy who did win that item got on stage and had a tough game, which he didn't end up winning. It was back to contestant's row and the final item bid of the day. I was nervous because I knew this was my last chance, and thought how much it would stink to get this far and then not get on that stage.

The next item for bid were pots and pans. I remember thinking, "Ok, now those I can use." The girl next to me bid $700. I was planning on bidding $700 though, so it took me a second to decide what my next move would be. I didn't want to be one of those "jerks" that bids $1 over what the last person did, so I decided that I would go with $750. I was the highest bidder. The total retail price for the pots and pans ended up being a little over $1300. Since I was the closest bidder without going over the price, Bob called me up on stage. I gave him the traditional kiss on the cheek. He had kind eyes and asked me a few questions about where I went to school and what year I was in, as he led into the big reveal of what I was going to be playing for…a brand new car!! I remember my stomach turning over and holding my breath as the doors opened and a brand new black Ford Escort station wagon (that's right I said a station wagon) was revealed.

This car, compared to my heater-less Plymouth, was like an incredible dream, shiny and black sitting on that stage. I remember praying and hoping that I would win because it would be such a bummer to get this far and lose.

The game that I played was "Pick a Pair". I had to pick a pair of products that had the same price. There were six items to choose from, and suddenly I had no idea how much items such as toothpaste, popcorn and stain remover cost. I looked nervously past the cameras in my face to my girlfriends who were screaming at the top of their lungs what they thought my choices should be. First, I chose the toothpaste. When the price revealed that it was $4.99, I remember thinking, "Gosh, toothpaste doesn't cost that much in Vermont"!

I was a little thrown at the price so I looked helplessly at the girls who were saying "the remover, the remover". I chose the remover, which had a price of $1.99. I thought it was all over, my chance was blown, but Bob looked at me and said I was going to have one more chance. I said, "Ok", and I know that at this point my heart was beating out of my chest and my head was whirling so fast. I had no idea what other product would match either price. Frantically I turned again to the girls. Now luckily for us, we happened to have sat in front of a group of sweet women from Canada, who had been watching the show and pricing items for the last year in anticipation of their attendance to a taping. They started telling my girlfriends which products to have me choose. I told Bob that I was going to get rid of the toothpaste and choose a product that was $1.99. He laughed at how matter of fact I was. The girls were screaming "popcorn" now like it was a life or death matter, so I shrugged my shoulders and nervously said "Popcorn?" The sign for the popcorn popped up as Bob said dramatically, "Is that popcorn $1.99, does she win that car…. Yes!!" The $1.99 lit up and I dropped to my knees with joy. Tears started welling up in my eyes, and as Bob put his arm around me and reiterated that this was MY car sitting on the "Price is Right" stage, I looked at those smiling blue eyes and said "Thank you SO much".

My exact thought at that exact moment was "I can't believe something good just happened." As I mentioned before, going on this trip came at one of the most traumatic points in my life, a time when it seemed like everything was going wrong, a time when I felt that what I should do was crawl into a hole where no one could see me, or run away from my current reality.

THIS moment changed everything. It changed my perspective. It didn't just change the perspective of my situation at school, or with my family drama, it changed my entire outlook on life. It was the moment that I BELIEVED that a small town girl from Vermont, who didn't know how to apply makeup, who had never traveled so far from home, and who had been shy for the majority of her life…COULD do anything. I believed in that moment that I was special and I believed with everything in me that I was destined for greatness. It was a moment where my confidence grew, dreams and goals suddenly seemed attainable and I realized that God had a huge plan for me and nothing was out of reach.

This moment would be a catalyst for me to overcome many of my own personal doubts and start making the changes and choices that would shape my future.

I was floating on a cloud that day as I left the studio. I had a chance to spin the big wheel, but my numbers went over $1.00 so I didn't get to the Showcase Showdown, and at that point I didn't care. I remember just wanting to desperately find the girls so that I could hug them and scream with them. As I was released from backstage after going over a bunch of paperwork and tax information, I excitedly ran outside. Along the way people were giving me high fives, saying "Hey Diana, will you give me a ride in your new car?"

I tried calling my Dad from the studio, but there were so many people screaming behind me that my Dad had no clue what I was saying, and actually thought something bad had happened! When I finally got in touch with him and the rest of my family, they were thrilled and couldn't believe that something so amazing had happened. This day was definitely one of the top ten most awesome days of my life.

I think up until this experience, fear really had a grip on me…fear of the unknown, fear of rejection, fear of failure. Even though my dreams and goals weren't directed towards the fitness industry at this point in time, I did know that I wanted to do something important. The lesson I learned was that if I ever wanted to achieve anything in life, I had to first believe that it was possible.

The most important lesson I hope you take away with you after reading this story, is that your ability to succeed at achieving a goal, whether it is weight loss and physical transformation, overcoming emotional hurts, or something else, starts in your mind. The start of your personal transformation has to start with that switch going on in your mind flicking from "I can't" to "I can".

As soon as you believe in yourself, you CAN achieve anything you set your mind to. You CAN find ways around any obstacle that steps in your way if you want something badly enough for yourself. I invite you to take a minute and think back to a time when you realized that you were great at something, when you realized you were special or capable, when you knew that you had been selling yourself short and you were far more capable than you ever realized.

Do you have some of those experiences? Do you believe that it's true? Have you had your own personal "ah-ha" moment? If you haven't, then perhaps right now, this very instant will be one for you. It doesn't take being on national television, or being in a car crash, or seeing yourself on the cover of a magazine to experience a powerful moment that will change your mind, change your thinking patterns, and change your life.

CHAPTER SIX
FROM FAT TO HITCH FIT

Diana's Story: Part 3

For the rest of my college career, I had a completely different outlook on life. I was now more excited to graduate and take on my future. I still had no idea what I wanted to do in life, but I wasn't afraid to try anything anymore. I wasn't afraid to travel. I wasn't afraid to think big.

Over the next few years, I went for dream after dream. (*If you are interested in reading my detailed memoir please be sure to pick up a copy of my Fitness Model E-book available summer 2011). In a nutshell, my endeavors included running for Miss Vermont USA (I placed 4th and realized that pageant world was NOT for me!) and working in a miserable office job that I hated with all my heart.

I finally had an epiphany that the gym was the one place that I LOVED to be, and that was the place I wanted to work every day in order to be happy. I quit the office job, moved to Utah, and started pursuing my dream of working in fitness. I received my certifications from ACE and AFAA, and also attended a 6-week vocational program for personal trainers and group fitness instructors in Maui, HI called Strong, Stretched and Centered. I learned more during that six week program than I could have possibly imagined, and it took my training to a completely different level while opening more opportunities for me.

Another big dream I had was to work as a fitness director on a cruise ship. I figured that would be the ultimate job since I loved to travel and I loved fitness. As I did my research, I found that cruise ship jobs were not so easy to come by, especially for Americans (deemed lazy by cruise ship standards). That didn't deter me.

The opportunity arose to apply for a cruise ship job while I was attending school in Maui, so I jumped at the chance. Five months after submitting my resume and application to Norwegian Cruise Lines, I received a phone call that, once again, would change the course of my life. They offered me the position of fitness director on one of their ships, which meant quitting my current job (I was working at a gym in Park City, Utah as a personal trainer and my little business was growing and thriving!), and just being ready to GO whenever they called. I didn't hesitate. I immediately prepared for this next adventure. Within a few short weeks, I was whisked away to Hawaii to begin working on my cruise adventure.

It was during this period of time, however, that physically, I took a turn for the worse. I still was very uneducated when it came to nutrition (despite all of my training certifications, I STILL had never been taught how to eat properly, and still had no idea how to change my body utilizing the food that I was eating). Despite the fact that I was teaching loads of fitness classes on the ship, the poor eating choices and alcohol consumption led to my gain of almost 30 pounds over the course of the year I was on the ship. That was the heaviest I had ever been in my life.

I remember standing on the scale on the ship, and was horrified to see it go up into the 170's. I quickly stepped off. That was the last time I would set foot on a scale for months. I was too terrified to see what it said. I was still full of excuses too. I blamed my weight gain on me getting older, on slow metabolism, on the fact that I was just becoming more "womanly". I refused to acknowledge that it was my own horrible, hidden eating behaviors that were causing the gain. You see, during this time, despite the fact that I was surrounded with people. I felt very sad and very lonely. The holidays hit me the worst. I was far away from home, with no family around, and even though I went out to celebrate with friends, I found that I was emotionally eating to soothe my unhappiness.

I got off the ship in February of 2004 and one of the first people I saw when I got off the ship was my little sister. She hadn't seen me for quite a while, and the look of shock on her face at my weight gain was enough to let me know I had let things go too far and it was time for a change.

While I was still on the cruise ship, I talked incessantly about wanting to one day compete in a Figure competition. The entire time I lived in Park City, I had talked about it non-stop too. I had posters of my favorite female competitors such as Maggie Diubaldo and Monica Brant plastered all over my walls during that time. I had been telling my friends that one day I would be in Oxygen magazine, and yet here I was, instead of being in better shape, I was in the worst condition I'd ever been in.

My clothes were tight. I hated what I saw when I looked in the mirror. I hated how sluggish and squishy my body felt. This was the worst I had ever looked or felt in my life. It crushed my self-confidence, and unfortunately that just led to even more poor eating behaviors. I found myself binge eating at night, when everyone else was asleep. I didn't want anyone to see what I was doing to myself and I even caught myself making statements about how confused I was that I wasn't losing weight.

I did drop a few pounds initially after getting off the ship, just because I wasn't consuming mass quantities of cruise ship food on a weekly basis. Still, my weight held fast in the upper 160's, and it wasn't going to budge until I made some major changes. I wasn't ready though so I kept procrastinating. I knew it was going to take a drastic change, but I wasn't ready to give up my current lifestyle.

It was almost like I was too sad and lonely to do it for myself yet. I didn't want to be judged. I wanted to be able to be the "fun" girl at the parties. I just wasn't ready to make a commitment to myself for the transformation to take place.

I ended up moving to San Antonio, Texas shortly after the cruise ship adventure. I lived with my sister Linda and her husband Scott. They took me into their home and gave me a place for a fresh start. After living there for a few months, I was FINALLY ready for my transformation to take place. I had completely run out of excuses, and I was so sick and tired of saying "someday I want to be in great shape", "someday I want to be in Oxygen". I finally realized that my "someday" was never going to come if I kept on making excuses. There was absolutely nothing holding me back from success except for myself.

I had a massive "ah-ha" moment on July 5, 2005. I was working at a gym in San Antonio when one of my fellow trainers came up to me and said, "What are you waiting for?" Well that did it. The light bulb went off in my head. I signed up for my first competition that day. I finally committed to change my eating habits THAT day. I made my life change THAT day. I didn't wait "till Monday". I didn't say "I'll start next week". I started literally THAT day. I found a trainer to kick my butt during workouts. I also found someone to help me with my nutrition since getting really lean for a show was going to require more than a regular weight loss program.

Over the course of the next 18 weeks, I didn't just transform my body. I transformed my life. I immediately started to see how changing my nutrition was changing my physique. I committed myself 100% to my program. I was the type who would not cheat on my plan if you paid me too. I just wouldn't do it. All I could think was that my butt was going to be on stage in a bikini, and people were going to be JUDGING it!!" Trust me. That was enough motivation for me to stay on course. No matter how long it took.

I found that along the way I did have to cut negatives out of my life. I found that people, who had been friends before, didn't want to hang out with me anymore because I wasn't "fun" anymore. I didn't care. I didn't miss the partying. I didn't miss feeling like garbage in the morning after a night of drinking. I felt like I was finally on the track that I was supposed to be on, and I didn't want anything to stand in my way.

When I finally stepped on stage in November 2005, I could absolutely say that I had done everything possible to be in the best shape for that day. I didn't look back and think, "Oh I slacked off here or there and could have done better." I knew I had given it my all, and now it was time for the big show. I ended up placing first, and it ignited something in me that I didn't know existed. I felt like I found IT. I had found my calling. I was supposed to be a part of this business. It was one of the most amazing feelings I had ever felt.

Over the course of the next four years, I went on to win 6 more titles including a World Champion Fitness Model title and WBFF Figure World Champion title. I earned my WBFF Pro status in 2008 and finally received my opportunity to do a photo shoot for the magazine I had always dreamed of being in, Oxygen.

Not only did going after my dreams lead to success within the industry that I love, it also led me to meet the love of my life, Micah LaCerte. Had it not been for this industry, Micah and I would have never crossed paths, and Hitch Fit would not be what it is today.

That is my story in a nutshell. My life hasn't been perfect, or anything close to being perfect. I have screwed up on a lot of things, and I've made my fair share of negative choices. Of that you can be sure. But the thing is, I'm entirely grateful for every choice, whether good or bad. I'm entirely grateful for every struggle. I'm glad that I struggled with my weight, that I experienced what it feels like to be uncomfortable in my own skin. I can appreciate the hard work that it takes to get in shape.

It's your turn. Your transformation begins inside. It begins with what you believe you are capable of. You have it in you to do whatever you want, so please go for it! Give it all you've got and never be afraid of falling. That is how you grow stronger…when you learn to pick yourself back up!

CHAPTER SEVEN
YOUR TRANSFORMATION =
INSPIRATION + PERSPIRATION

This book is about transformation. Our goal is to show you how you can transform your physical appearance. Even more than that, however, we want to teach you how to **completely** transform your lifestyle so that you not only look great on the outside, but also feel great on the inside, and have a stronger sense of happiness and fulfillment with your life. This will be a mind, body and soul transformation.

We will share with you the keys to making positive choices in your life on a daily basis that will ultimately allow you to achieve your goals. What you have to understand is that while we are your guides and motivators, YOU are the one that has to put this in motion in your life. YOU are the one that has to make the commitment. YOU are the one who has to make the right choices day in and day out to get to where you want to be.

You and only you possess the power and responsibility to make the change that you desire happen. When you accept that fact fully, and take ownership of it, you CAN achieve anything you set your mind to.

Before we go any further, we want to make a promise to you. We will be 100% honest in the information that we share with you. Our goal is to give you the truth about weight loss…to really educate you about your body. We aren't interested in lying to you about how easy weight loss will be. We aren't interested in telling you that it's only going to take 3 minutes a day on some machine to get six pack abs and the body of your dreams.

We aren't going to tell you that what we've achieved with our own physiques only took a little bit of work and a magic pill. We are serious about what we do in this industry, and we want to go to sleep at night with a clear conscience, knowing that we shared the best knowledge we could, and provided the best tools for people to actually be successful. Lying to you, or suggesting a quick fix isn't going to help anyone. So, as we continue, rest assured that we are here to help and will always be honest, even at the cost of it being brutal.

Most of the fitness and weight loss advertising you hear out there is a big fraud. We detest all of the false information and false weight loss advertising we are bombarded with on a daily basis. It seems everywhere you look there is another ad for a miracle pill or magic potion or new fad diet that is going to get you a phenomenal six pack set of abs, so it's really no wonder that most people have no clue what it takes to transform their bodies.

You are told so many **lies**:

- It's easy;

- It takes only a small commitment;

- You can do it without eating right and exercising; or

- You can have an amazing physique without changing any of your current habits.

We are bombarded with misleading messages on television, the

Internet, in magazines, on the radio. You get the point.

Here's the real deal. Transformation is NOT easy. Changing habits in your life that have been established for months, years or even decades, is hard work. It doesn't happen overnight, and it doesn't happen as drastically as it does on shows like "The Biggest Loser" (unless you quit your job, leave your family, work out for 6 to 8 hours per day, and eat an extremely low calorie diet that will also cause an awful lot of muscle waste at the same time).

Did you know that many testimonials you see on infomercials or in ads are PAID testimonials? That's right. The person on the ad may not have, and in many instances, probably did NOT use the product or contraption they are promoting to get their weight loss results. What they likely did, instead, was lose the weight via diet and exercise, got some killer before and after pictures, and then were offered money from product companies allowing their pictures to be used as testimonials. This happens ALL the time.

You are being misled on a daily basis, which is why the fitness and diet industry is a multi-billion dollar industry with an extremely high failure rate. When the ads have the microscopic "results not typical" verbiage down at the bottom of their ads, they aren't kidding! There is nobody in this world with a great body and sexy abs who hasn't worked hard to attain them.

These people have made choices and sacrifices in order to achieve their fitness goals. They have worked hard, eaten properly, and trained their booties off. Ignore all the fraudulent fitness claims out there. BE skeptical of anything that seems too easy, or claims to have amazing results with little time and little work. If it sounds too good to be true, then it likely IS too good to be true. Follow what we are going to share with you, and you will see results on the outside - and more importantly, on the inside.

One of the greatest things about Hitch Fit is that when you make the changes, follow the plan, and take responsibility for your choices, results ARE typical. We don't need to put fine print under our before and after stories (to see Hitch Fit before and after pictures, videos and testimonials, log on to www.hitchfit.com). We don't have people saying how simple and easy it was to change their lives. In fact, the majority of them will be perfectly honest about how hard it was, and how they went through struggles and overcame obstacles to achieve their own personal transformations. That's the good stuff - the truth. That's the stuff that changes lives. That's the stuff we want to share with you so that you too can experience this powerful change and start leading your best life.

This transformation process is split up into three categories: lifestyle, fitness and nutrition. The key is to achieve balance in these three areas so you can:

- Eliminate your insecurities;

- Set and accomplish your goals;

- Lead a more effective and efficient life;

- Eliminate negativity; and

- Reach a higher level of physical, mental, emotional and spiritual health and happiness.

This plan possesses a "Pay it Forward" attitude. Once your

transformation is complete and you have achieved your own personal version of success, we encourage you to share your story. When you reach that place, you have the unique opportunity to tell your tale of overcoming adversity and obstacles. At this point, YOU become the inspiration for others struggling with similar situations.

You see, since every person is different and everyone has a unique story, YOUR particular story is going to be one that someone out there can really relate too. Not everyone is going to be able to relate to one of our stories, or even to one of our current transformation stories, but it may be YOUR journey, YOUR experience, that they read about once your transformation is complete, that allows them to experience their very own "ah-ha" moment, that will be their catalyst for change. YOU may be the reason that someone down the road makes the choices that will save their life resulting in a higher quality, happier and more productive life. How cool is that?

CHAPTER EIGHT
LIFESTYLE: KEYS TO HAPPINESS

What do you think the majority of people want most in life? In this line of work, after interacting with thousands of people, the number one desire that we hear is that people want to be happy. Personal happiness is subjective, but in general we believe that it is an overall feeling of satisfaction and joy with who you are, what you do and your place in this world.

We believe you can achieve overall happiness in all areas of your life, including your physical, mental, emotional, spiritual and financial states of being, by completing the following steps:

- Eliminate negativity from your life;
- Focus on the positive;
- Have a strong spiritual belief system;
- Confront sources of emotional pain;
- Discover what your passion in life is; and,
- Give back from the gifts with which you have been blessed.

Eliminate Negativity

Every single one of us has a story. That is one of the reasons we love getting to know people. On the outside, many people appear to be fine, carefree and happy, but on the inside they are struggling. Everyone has suffered through something in their life, and that something has had a major part in shaping them into the person they are today. Everyone has faced situations that were difficult and challenging.

Some of these situations were controllable and some were uncontrollable. Some people have suffered through disease, death of family and friends, injuries, divorce, abusive physical, sexual or emotional relationships, financial distress, just to name a few of the most common. Some people come out of these challenges being better people and leading positive, happy and productive lives, while some people get so stuck in the negativity of the situation that they are completely controlled by it and end up constantly living in a state of unhappiness. Why does this happen?

It all boils down to the choices we make. We all possess the power and the responsibility to make the right choices in our lives. If you choose to make positive choices that enhance the quality and quantity of your life, you will be on the right path toward that desired state of waking up in the morning happy to be alive and loving your purpose and place in the world.

We are all broken people in some way, shape or form. We both are, and every single person either of us have encountered in life has been hurt or damaged in some way, by someone, or some situation. But guess what, we've news for you though; you don't have to let your past or even current situation have control over your life anymore. You absolutely have the power to change the course of your life.

The first step in taking charge of that power is to cut out all the negativity from your life. Negativity can come in a wide variety of shapes and forms, including: alcohol, drugs, food addictions, abusive relationships that you stay in, and unhealthy environments or situations that you continue to put yourself in. Anything controllable that is dragging you into a state of depression or self-pity must be eliminated from your life in order to find yourself, to get yourself back, and to love living life again.

Cut out the negative. Sounds simple doesn't it? Not necessarily. Negativity can be addictive, and in a lot of cases you actually feel like you NEED that negative influence in your life. If you can reach the moment where you break free, though…when you can just let go…you will feel an incredible weight lifted from your shoulders. It is then that you will experience the freedom to pursue a brighter and more fulfilling future.

Here are some steps to take to eliminate negative situations, thoughts or even people from your life. Taking these actions can allow you to experience an energizing freedom that may be totally foreign to you right now. Get out a pen and paper and take a good hard look at yourself, at your current situation, and at the things that are bringing you down or holding you back.

Now some of your "negatives" are uncontrollable, and some WILL be controllable. It's important to recognize the things that you do have the ability to make alternate choices about, and make change happen. You're going to have to take ACTION for any change to occur. So, once you have had the time to go over your list, it is time to work on HOW you intend to change your current situation to make room for the more positive choices to have their maximum impact.

Here is a list of questions to get you started in the right direction. Feel free to add more of your own if they come to you.

1. What situations do you find yourself in where you are tempted to or are consistently making poor choices? Are these situations that can be avoided? If yes, then what will your alternate situation be?

2. What are your playgrounds? Where do you spend a lot of your time? Is spending time in these places allowing you to progress toward your goals of becoming more physically, spiritually, emotionally or financially fit? If it isn't a place that is helping you progress in one of these areas, it is probably an environment you don't need to be spending time in. What other

environment would be a better alternative, and a more positive place for you to start working towards your goals?

3. What are your strongholds? Do you have an addiction to something that you need to let go of? Perhaps in order to drown out emotional pain or to relieve stress, you are turning to alcohol or drugs, or to a tub of ice cream in the wee hours of the morning or to a box of chocolates. What is your strategy for eliminating these strongholds? Perhaps by avoiding the situations where these temptations are present is a good start!

4. What relationships are detrimental to your physical, spiritual or emotional well-being? Do you have friends or family members who put you down on a regular basis in order to make themselves feel better? Do you have people in your life who tell you that you can't achieve your goals, who try to pressure you to do things that are negative or who abuse you in some way? Are these people that you can end communication with, or spend less time with? What would be the worst thing to happen if you ended a negative relationship in your life?

This next one, (5) please do on a separate piece of paper. The negative thoughts that you allow to pervade your mind on a daily basis set you up for failure from the beginning. If you tell yourself that you "can't" do something, then you are absolutely right. Vice versa, if you tell yourself you "CAN" do something, then again, you are absolutely right. Your first step towards achieving your goals in all other areas is by believing in yourself, and that starts with eliminating the negative thoughts from your mind. When you are finished writing out all the negatives you are telling yourself, then it is time to throw those negatives away. Literally! **Tear up the sheet of paper, or even burn it if you can do that without burning your house down!** *Whatever you do, get rid of it and use that as a symbol of eliminating those thoughts that are controlling your destiny now.*

47

5. What are the negative thoughts that you repeat to yourself on a regular basis? What are you telling yourself that you believe is true? Do you say that you "can't"? That you aren't good enough? That you aren't strong enough? That you have failed in the past, so you will probably fail now too? Do you tell yourself you're not worth it? List out every negative thought you have found floating through your mind. Get it out right now. Every single thing that you write on this paper is **NOT TRUE** of you. It is not the real you. You are capable of so much more. Now, destroy the paper. This is not your reality. It is time to take steps towards the new you.

Once you have compiled the list of negatives you must deal with, it's time to come up with a plan of action. You have some tough choices and some sacrifices to make in order to gain or regain control of your life.

Now, we're not saying that eliminating negative relationships and environments from your life is going to be easy, and we're not saying that the answer is necessarily to instantly cut people out of your life, but you do have to confront the situation if you want it to change.

For example, let's say you have a friend who leads a crazy lifestyle… partying, drinking, or doing drugs… and is constantly pressuring you to join in the "fun." Maybe you have gone along with it for a while as a way to deal with personal issues, but you have had enough and are ready to get your mojo back, or get your business back on track or start filling your life with positive relationships.

You need to have a crucial conversation with this person and explain to them where you are and make them aware of the journey you plan to embark on. See how they respond. If they are a true friend, they are going to support you and stop trying to get you involved with negative activities. If they still want to pressure you and disrespect your choice, you need to cut that negativity out of your life.

In some instances, these are people you will need to let go from your life for good. In other cases, it may be just for a short time until you can get back on track. When the negative people in your life are family members, a spouse or a girlfriend or boyfriend, the situation can be even more difficult. If you really seek to become the best person you can be, you must communicate with each person, and regardless of your relationship, limit your contact with them while you learn how to interact with them in a constructive way.

A boyfriend or girlfriend who is holding you back or putting you down is probably not the person that you should be with, and you must find it within yourself to let them go. If it is your spouse, seek counseling or the services of an organization that can help you change that negative relationship into a positive one.

When you have identified the negative influences in your life, do not procrastinate to eliminate them. Life is way too short for you to continue living in negativity when there are so many positive people and experiences out there waiting for you. What can you do today, right now, that is going to get you one step closer to where you want to be? Figure out what that is and just do it! Maybe it's a workout, maybe it's getting rid of junk food in your house, maybe it is breaking up with a boyfriend or girlfriend, and maybe it is staying sober for the night. Whatever it is, TODAY IS THE DAY TO START MAKING THE CHANGE!

Focusing on the Positive

The next thing you need to do is make a list of the positive people, places and things in your life. You know the negatives that you have to cut out. In their place, you need to surround yourself with positive influences and put your focus and emphasis into those. Surround yourself with positive people and friends. Get involved with a group or activity that will be a positive force in your life. This could be a support group, a church group, a social network such as the Hitch Fit online community or a sport or physical activity.

Get out there, make some new friends who have similar goals as you, people who will support you and push you to excel. There are people out there willing to lend a hand and when you look for them you will find them. Every time either of us have reached a low in life and needed a helping hand, when we looked, sure enough there was someone there to reach out to. Look around you, those people who can be positive forces in your life are there. Get involved and get connected with these types of people. When you surround yourself with positive people, places and situations, you will find it will make you a more positive and happy person too.

The key to making lasting change and ultimately being the happiest you are able, is to start making positive and productive choices on a daily basis in every aspect of your life. When you look at yourself in the mirror or review your current emotional, mental, spiritual or financial state, you have a choice to make.

Let's say you are very dissatisfied with what you look like physically. You can whine and complain about your current state of being, or you can say "Hey, I've let myself go over the last couple of years. I've been through hardships and I've made my share of excuses. All of that is in the past now, and I have a bright future ahead of me. Now is the time for change. Now is the time for me to get in the best shape ever, set realistic goals for myself and make the right choices every day so I will be able to look in this mirror and feel proud of the reflection staring back at me."

The final step to focus on the positives is to write out NEW thoughts, positive affirmations that you need to read to yourself on a daily basis. As we said before, this change has got to begin in your mind, by believing in yourself. The first step to believing is to tell yourself every day how capable you are. It doesn't matter if you read these words right now and don't fully believe them. If you read them enough on a regular basis, you WILL start to believe them. Here are just a few ideas of what you can say about YOU!

> - I am fit.
> - I am strong.
> - I am healthy and happy.
> - I wake up every day with a smile on my face.
> - I make healthy eating choices and I love doing it!
> - I make time for myself.
> - I love to exercise.
> - I look in the mirror and love the way I look and feel.
> - I have the job of my dreams as an _____.
> - I am financially sound and make _____ per year.
> - I am so in love and with the woman/man of my dreams.
> - My belief system is strong.
> - I have faith that I am a special person with a specific purpose.

You can of course expand on this, change it, make it yours. But keep it all positive and keep it all present tense. Avoid saying "I will be happy." Start telling your mind right now that you ARE happy, that you ARE successful. It doesn't matter that it may not be true at this exact moment. When you tell your mind something, it will aid you in finding a way to make it your reality.

As we mentioned before, we've all had challenges, struggles and negative things that have happened in our lives. You can choose to allow these things to make you a stronger and better person. When people see the success we have personally experienced, they make the mistaken assumption that the road has been an easy one, that life didn't throw curveballs, and all things were just handed over freely.

We can assure you, that we have had plenty of mountains to climb, tragedies to overcome, and abuses to heal. The road has been anything but easy in reaching this place in life, and honestly… the journey, the growing, the healing never ends. It's a constant process until the day we die. Although Micah loves to joke and say "I came out of the womb this way," it has been a very hard road. However, by making positive choices, eliminating negativity, and trusting God that His way was the best way, we both have come to believe that success is possible in all aspects…despite what life has to throw at us!

Develop a strong belief system

When it comes to being happy on a regular basis, hands down, the main reason for the greatest sense of fulfillment in our personal lives is based around our belief in God. We are both born-again Christians, believing that Jesus Christ is the son of God and that He came to earth to shed his blood for our sins. We believe that we are His children. We believe that we are completely imperfect, yet He loves us still and always will. We believe that He has an incredible purpose for our lives, and the main goal for us is to fulfill that to the best of our abilities.

Having this deep sense of connection with our Creator enables us to see His hand working in our lives, and see a bigger picture and reason for everything that we do! Even though our job is about the "physical" side of things, we both absolutely know that this is only one small piece of the puzzle. We know that these physical bodies will deteriorate and age, and are only a temporary place to live. We are utterly convinced, though, that it is our responsibility to take care of them and treat them with respect while we reside in them. True happiness, deep happiness, doesn't come from landing a magazine cover. It comes from knowing that you are a unique creation, completely special in and of yourself, utterly loved by the One who made you, and that there is a deep purpose for your life that only you can fulfill.

We aren't here to preach at you, but it's an actual proven truth that people with strong belief systems are more deeply satisfied and happier in their lives than those who flounder through life not believing in anything. We wanted to share our beliefs with you because they truly are a huge part of why we do what we do, why we are the way we are, why we make the choices that we make, and why we are so happy with the path laid before us.

As you embark on this journey, let it not just be one in the physical. If you don't have a solid belief system, then we encourage you to start seeking truth, and start discovering the state of your spiritual health and being. Being in the best shape of your life, or having a lot of material possessions, will never fulfill you completely. If you go through the physical transformation, but don't delve into the spiritual side of things, there will always be something missing, and you will still be seeking that empty piece of the puzzle.

A couple of great resources for spiritual growth (these are all NON denominational, so it doesn't matter what religion you are) include, but are not limited to: Max Lucado. He is an amazing teacher and you will learn a lot from his straight forward, easy to read books and teachings. His website is www.maxlucado.com and you can actually tune in to see broadcasts live from Oak Hills Church in San Antonio on Sundays at www.oakhillschurchsa.org. Another great resource for ladies is Women of Faith www.womenoffaith.com. Their conferences are AMAZING. They have women's conferences and ones for teenage girls. The conferences are held at various locations nationwide. And finally, Beth Moore is awesome. She has a great selection of Bible studies, some of which can be done online. You will learn so much about how special you are to God through this woman's work. You can find out more about Beth at www.lifeway.com. Remember that these are just some of the resources available. They are ones that have helped us in our journey and we offer the information here to give you a place to start.

Confront Sources of Emotional Pain

We've said this a few times now. Everyone has a story. We've all had something to overcome in our lives. Some have dealt with it in ways that led to positives. Some, however, have chosen the alternate route and allowed these trials and tribulations to lead to negative and unhealthy choices, that are now directly affecting their very health and quality of living.

We work with a lot of people who are struggling with their weight due to having succumbed to emotional eating. You may be one of these people and may very well be able to relate to exactly the scenario we are about to describe. Emotional eaters turn to food for comfort, to fill a void if they are sad or lonely or stressed or depressed or happy or wanting to celebrate. Regardless of the situation, the thought of food and the desire for food pervades the majority of their thoughts. There is a brief, very brief, feeling of comfort that comes from consuming whatever the craving is calling for. Often times this behavior is done in secret.

Emotional eaters tend to hide their behavior. They may go all day without eating much where people can see them, and then later in the evening or when they are home alone, they consume massive amounts of calories in short periods of time. Emotional eaters have a high tendency of saying that they can't control their eating, and that diets don't work. They are often in denial about the quantity of food they are eating. They typically have a sense of being out of control of this aspect of their lives and thus are incredibly unhappy.

This type of behavior is stemming from somewhere. There is usually a root to the problem. There is something within that this behavior is attempting to heal or soothe. Emotional eaters may claim that they "just love to eat", but that is typically not the truth...there is usually something eating them instead. Tony Robbins has a wonderful way of explaining the reason why emotional eaters do what they do. In his "pain versus pleasure" philosophy (which you can read about in his books "Unlimited Power" or "Unleash the Power Within"). Basically the emotional eater is attaching a great deal of pleasure to the act of eating, to the physical act of putting food in their mouth, chewing it up and swallowing it, and then to the brief, very brief feeling of euphoria that follows eating high fat or high sugar foods. The act of emotional eating is thought of as a source of pleasure, as opposed to the source of pain which it actually is. However, long term effects of these actions include:

o *the scale going up,*
o *body fat increasing,*
o *self esteem decreasing,*
o *the decreased ability to use your body the way it was intended,*
o *energy levels decreasing,*
o *health deteriorating,*
o *development of diseases such as diabetes, high blood pressure,*

high cholesterol and more,
- *the inability to wear the clothes that you want to wear,*
- *the inability to keep up with your kids,*
- *lack of energy to be the best parent, boyfriend, girlfriend, or spouse that you can be.*

These are all painful things, not things that are pleasurable. And all of these consequences can stem from the act of emotional eating. It's really not that pleasurable when you really think about what you are actually doing to your body.

The euphoric feeling that comes immediately after emotional eating is often followed very closely by feelings of self-loathing and guilt. Not only that, but this behavior is what sets you, your body, and your health up for disaster. It's a vicious cycle that CAN stop if you decide to take the power and gain control over the situation. Now, that may be easier than it sounds. However, the bottom line is the only one who controls your behaviors, who makes the choice to take a food, put it in your mouth and eat it, is you and only you. For most of you, the one who makes the choices at the grocery store as far as what to purchase and place in your fridge for consumption, is YOU. The only one who makes the decision to stop at the fast food restaurant on the way to or from work, or both, is YOU. These are all actions that you can put a stop to. If you want something badly enough, there is a way to achieve it!

We know that overcoming emotional eating is not going to be easy, so here are some ideas on how to start this process. The absolute first thing you have to do is get the junk out of your house. Literally **throw it away**, or if you feel bad about throwing it away, donate it to a homeless shelter or soup kitchen. Regardless, get it OUT of your house. Don't think "I'll just finish what's left in this container". NO. Throw it away now. That junk, whatever it may be, whether it's cookies, candy, soda, chips, fast food, etc. is sabotage. It will not help you get one step closer to your goal. In fact, it will more than likely set you back.

Every time you make the choice to give in to it, you are saying **that** instant, **that** moment when the food goes into your mouth and down your throat, is **MORE important** to you than your fitness, your health and possibly even the ultimate goal of taking your life back. If you don't have those foods in your house and within easy reach, you are far less likely to go to the store and purchase them when you get a craving.

The next step is to start a journal. You have to start recognizing the emotions you feel when you have the urge to eat foods that are destroying your body and your health. When you have a craving, if you can just deter yourself for about 10 to 15 minutes, instead of giving in to it immediately, a lot of times the craving will go away. Imagine the awesome feeling you will have knowing that you made a good choice for yourself! A good way to distract yourself is to keep your journal handy. Rather than pacing back and forth in front of the refrigerator saying "will I" or "won't I" (because that is a losing battle), get your journal, sit down and start writing. Be sure that you have your goals (and a reminder such as a picture) of your goals, visible in that journal and handy. Having your "before" pictures pasted in there is highly recommended too. Those pictures can be very powerful motivators if you are truly serious about changing your body and your life!

While you are writing in that journal, you also need to take some time for self-reflection, being honest about where the hurts, disappointments and pain are from. We have heard so many people, totally broken by the trials and struggles they have been handed in this life. Some of these include: being abandoned at childhood by a parent; being sexually abused or physically abused; experiencing the death of a parent, or a child; a painful divorce or breakup; losing a loved one to cancer or some other horrible illness; or suffering through an illness personally. The list can go on and on.

Open up and let your heart spill onto the pages. Don't even think about what you're writing, just let it come out. These are your personal and private thoughts. You don't have to share them with anyone. You may just be amazed - if you let that pen go and take on a mind of it's own, you may discover some things about yourself that you didn't even know.

If you have experienced truly traumatic things in your past, it is wise to also seek counseling. We aren't therapists, but we know the value of therapy and having someone help you through difficult emotions, thoughts and feelings that have been holding you back. Your freedom may come in the form of forgiving someone who hurt you (you don't even have to tell them you forgive them, just do it in your heart). You may need to let go of a situation that was out of your control and forgive YOURSELF for something. How you deal with the source of this emotional pain is up to you, but you MUST deal with it. If you don't deal with the root of the problem, then the consequences surfacing in the form of emotional eating (which in turn leads to being overweight and obese), will never permanently change.

Another action you can take if you are someone who tends to stop by fast food restaurants on a regular basis, is to find a new route to work or to school. Completely avoid driving past the source of your temptation. In some cases that may not be possible, especially if you live in a small town, but a big percentage of you can figure out an alternate route.

Advertising now is so powerful that just by seeing certain restaurant signage can trigger a "Pavlov's dog effect" and have your mouth watering for the disgusting garbage food that is televised on fast food commercials being eaten by skinny models who in reality probably never touch the stuff.

A great book to read about this topic containing a ton of information about how fast "food" isn't even real, but rather is a pile of processed mush that our bodies barely recognize as nourishment, is "The End of Overeating" by David A. Kessler, MD. We highly recommend it, especially if you are an emotional eater.

Identify if you have a Secret Sabotage Behavior

We say "secret" because a lot of times these sabotage behaviors are things people don't do when others are around or watching. Perhaps that is because we know these behaviors are detrimental to our fitness success but don't want to admit it. The first step to overcoming a personal sabotage behavior is identifying it. Here are a few of the classic cases of eating habits that can hold you back from achieving your weight loss goals.

- *Sabotage 1*: The "Mindless Snacker". These people typically snack continually throughout the day. A little taste here, a treat there, a bit of this and a nibble of that can add up to a LOT of extra calories at the end of the day. But since you didn't eat them seated at the table as a "meal" maybe you didn't count those calories into your daily total. The "Mindless Snacker" may not even realize that they are eating all day. One of the best tools for making a "Mindless Snacker" more accountable is an eating journal. If you struggle with this snacking behavior, write down everything that you eat throughout the day. When you can see it down on paper, it's not such a secret anymore.

- *Sabotage 2*: The "Evening Eater". Now this one I know many of you can relate to. Maybe you are one of millions who succumb to boredom eating in the evenings. It's very possible that you make healthy choices all day long, but when you are lounging on the couch unwinding in the evenings, the urge to start munching gets the best of you. You may be consuming more calories during these late evening binges than you do all day. The "Evening Eater" usually isn't hungry. There is just the urge to have "something" while relaxing at the end of the day. You may not only be consuming excessive calories, but since your metabolism slows down at the end of the day, you won't be able to use all of those calories for energy. So, you guessed it, they will be stored as fat. My tips for the "Evening Eater" are to eat plenty of veggies at your evening meal so you will feel full. As soon as you finish your last meal of the day, brush your teeth or pop in a piece of sugar free gum so that you will be less tempted to eat again. If you feel that you must have something, drink some tea or flavored water. Drinking low calorie or no calorie drinks such as these will help to fill you up and decrease your urge to eat more.

- *Sabotage 3*: The "Starve and Stuff". These people typically don't eat breakfast. They don't eat much of anything for as long as they possibly can. But then it happens…around early afternoon they are so hungry they can't stand it any longer. At this point, their chance of making a healthy food choice is pretty much out the window. We've all been there before, those times when you're so hungry you can hardly even think, so you just fill yourself with whatever you can find. Usually this leads to overeating since it takes 15 to 20 minutes for your body to let you know it's full, and this little binge could result in hundreds, even thousands of calories in a very short period of time. If you eat this way, you will be on an energy roller coaster. Your resting metabolism rate will decrease. Your body will probably think you are starving, and when you eat mass amounts of calories it will hold onto them as fat. The best thing to do to avoid sabotaging yourself in this way is to eat consistently throughout the day, starting with breakfast. It is so important to eat this first meal in order to fire up your metabolism. Eat small snacks or meals every 2-3 hours throughout the day. When you do this, you won't ever feel like you are starving and you will be less likely to stuff yourself.

If you are struggling with a secret sabotage behavior, the first thing to do is recognize it! No matter how much you are exercising, if you are sabotaging your nutrition with these unhealthy eating habits you will never see the results that you desire. Take charge of those secret behaviors today and stop holding yourself back from fitness success.

Find Your Passion

One of the major pieces of the happiness puzzle is determining your passion in life. What were you placed on this earth to do? There are a million things you could be passionate about doing, so sit down and make a list. Some people are passionate about selling things, some about buying things, some love to write, some love to read, some like to organize, some like to clean, some like to care for others, some like to fix things, some like to teach, some like to learn, some like to listen, some like to speak, some love children, some love nature and the outdoors or animals. This list could go on and on, but you get the picture.

Do you enjoy the work that you currently do? Do you wake up happy in the morning and excited for your day? For us, it is working in the fitness industry and helping others. We wake up happy every single morning knowing that this is what we get to spend our time doing. If you can't say the same thing, then it's time to do some soul searching. The things you are passionate about are often going to be the things you are very good at doing. People with jobs or careers related to fields they are passionate about have a higher level of satisfaction and happiness and wake up every morning with a sense of purpose. If you aren't passionate about what you spend the majority of your time doing, then you need to make a change. Life is too short to continue on in a passionless environment.

Once you have discovered your passion, find ways to spend more of your time engaging in that activity. Oftentimes you will find that when you do what you are passionate about, you will find ways to make money doing it. Don't get me wrong - money is certainly not the way to happiness. Some of the wealthiest people we know are also some of the unhappiest people, so never assume that happiness comes hand in hand with financial success. If you can't find happiness when you are poor, you won't find it by getting rich. Waking up with a passion and purpose is one of the keys to happiness in life, whether you are a trash man or a cover model.

The bottom line is this: enjoy your life. We only have one to live, so make the most of it. Live in the present moment and take time to smell the roses. We fail to notice the joy and beauty in the little things because we are so busy and constantly looking toward what will happen in the future instead of realizing that we are living our life right now - this second - this is it.

We take the present for granted and forget that the future is not a promise. In an instant, our life could take a 180-degree turn. Be thankful for the things you do have and stop focusing on the things that you don't have. Live each day to the fullest, focus on the positive and live a life filled with passion.

Give Back

We think one of the greatest ways to experience happiness in your life is to give back to others. When you have been handed a challenge or obstacle in life and you overcome it, you automatically have a success story. Maybe your success was physical or financial, spiritual or emotional. Regardless of what area of life you achieved that success, you have an opportunity to help someone else who is struggling in that area. When you were in the midst of your struggle, certain people came into your life, perhaps just for a moment or a season, but those people had a hand in the victory over your challenge or in the healing process that followed.

You can share your experiences and how you overcame a challenge with someone who is going through a similar situation to let them know there is a light at the end of the tunnel.

There are so many ways you can give back that you may not even think of, and it's important to remember that a small effort on your part can have a major impact on the life of your friends, family, co-workers or even a stranger. You can share something as simple as a smile or an encouraging word. You can give of yourself emotionally by lending an ear to a friend who needs someone to listen, or mentally by educating someone on a topic they are unfamiliar with. You can give back to others financially by donating money to the cause of your choice.

You may encounter someone who has allowed themselves to deteriorate physically. Share your experience of getting yourself back to a state of physical fitness and offer to be a workout partner to someone in need of inspiration. The more you give of yourself to others the happier and more blessed you will be. When you pay that kindness forward and give of yourself to someone else, you will experience heart-felt joy and happiness.

One of our favorite ways to give back has been through sponsoring children in Haiti. It is a wonderful feeling to know that you are having a great impact on the life of someone you have never even met! If you are interested in sponsoring a child, one legit organization is World Vision www.worldvision.org. The other (which some of our family actually works with first hand and visits our children - so we know they are doing well and receiving the funds sent) is Monadnock Bible Conference and their Bridges of Love program. You can find out more information at www.monadnockbible.org . You can also get involved locally. Do searches for local homeless shelters, battered women's shelters, feeding programs, Boys and Girls Clubs, Big Brothers Big Sisters, or any number of other programs where you can get involved and make a major difference in someone's life.

CHAPTER NINE
MOTIVATION AND TRANSFORMATION

Underlying Motivation

You want a transformation. That's the main reason you are reading this book and participating in the Hitch Fit program. You are ready to make the necessary changes to your lifestyle and habits in order to finally reach your goals. Regardless of the type of transformation you are seeking or the areas of life you want to improve, there is one major question you must answer in order to begin your journey to a more fit, happy, healthy and successful version of you. What is your underlying motivation?

The first time we sit down with a new client, this is one of the first questions asked of them: Why? If you don't know what your motivation is, you are setting yourself up for failure. Changing your body and your life is a process. It doesn't happen overnight, and there are going to be challenges and obstacles along the way. In order to stay strong and focused with your eye on the prize, you must know WHY you are doing all of this to begin with. What is driving you to succeed? When your transformation is complete, what is it that you will have personally attained or achieved for yourself?

Your next step in this process is to write down what your main motivators are. The reason you have come to us for guidance could be a number of things. Maybe you are unhappy with what you see when you look in the mirror. Perhaps you are insecure in your relationship with your significant other. Tragically, your health may be in jeopardy or you've suffered a major life trauma and need to get back on your feet. Take a look through the following list of possible motivators and see if you can identify with any of them or come up with your own.

I want to….
- ✓ Have more energy and be more alert;
- ✓ Improve my mental focus and be more productive at work and at home;
- ✓ Be proud of what I see when I look in the mirror;
- ✓ Feel confident and have a healthier self image;
- ✓ Be healthy and get off medication;
- ✓ Be a good role model for my children and family members;
- ✓ Be a healthier person overall so that I don't develop diseases related to being overweight or obese;
- ✓ Strengthen my immune system;
- ✓ Feel more relaxed and less stressed out or anxious;
- ✓ Feel and look younger;
- ✓ Have a healthier and more active sex life with my partner;
- ✓ Be stronger so that I can keep up with my children;
- ✓ Improve my health so that I can have children;
- ✓ Feel like I am attractive to my significant other;
- ✓ Have more stamina to cope with my busy lifestyle;
- ✓ Build lean muscle tissue and feel more confident about myself;
- ✓ Fit into the cute clothes I want to wear;
- ✓ Improve my strength and fitness for a sport;
- ✓ Improve my balance and coordination;
- ✓ Sleep better;
- ✓ Improve my mood and reduce depression;
- ✓ Be a happier person and enjoy my life;
- ✓ Get to a place where I am physically, mentally, spiritually and emotionally happy;
- ✓ Be proud of who I am and what I do in this world;
- ✓ Fulfill a dream of competing in a fitness competition.

Once you have written down your underlying motivation, you need to keep it in a place where you are reminded of it on a daily basis. If your motivation is to fit into a smaller clothing size, hang up an article of clothing you would like to eventually wear, somewhere you can see it every single day. If your motivation is to be a good example to your children, keep a picture of them posted with a copy of your written motivation. If it is to get back to a weight that you were five years ago, post a picture of yourself from back then in a spot where you can see it.

Your motivation must be the first thing on your mind when you wake up in the morning. It has to be constantly present in your thoughts because you are going to be faced with temptations and choices on a daily basis. That motivator is what is going to keep you on track when these obstacles arise.

For example, let's say you are trying to lose 50 pounds of body fat because you are self-conscious about the way you look in your clothes. You want to improve your confidence level so you are more successful at work and in your personal relationships. You go out to eat with friends and make a healthy selection for the main course that will not throw you off track with your fitness goals, but then the dessert tray comes around and, wouldn't you know it, they have your favorite. It looks so good and smells so delicious, and everyone else is getting dessert, so why can't you?

This is where what is motivating you to make changes comes into play. You have worked incredibly hard with your workouts all week, and in this one piece of dessert you will erase an entire day of progress toward your goals, not to mention the lasting guilt you will feel after consuming it. It's a temporary indulgence that is simply not worth it in the big picture of attaining your goals. So, ask yourself, is it more important to eat the dessert and get a moment's satisfaction from the taste or is it more important to lose the weight that has been holding you back from the personal and professional success you desire?

The choice is yours. It's up to you to make the right one. Does this mean you can never have a cheat meal? Of course not, but throughout your transformation process it is very important to stay on track. The fewer lapses you have, the more quickly you will achieve your goals.

Once your transformation is complete and your body is in a maintenance phase, you will be able to enjoy your favorite treats and cheat meals on occasion and in moderation.

When you are faced with a temptation or situation such as this, keep your thought process positive. We promise you will feel good about making the healthy choice both on the outside and on the inside. What we mean by this is you can sit there and say "no" to dessert and then sulk at how you feel deprived and how you aren't able to enjoy something you really like, or you can switch the gears in your mind and focus on how proud you are of the choice you just made. You want to lose weight and be more confident with yourself, so you say no to dessert today because your body fat is currently at 30% (for example). Throughout your transformation you are going to reduce your body fat to 17% (for example).

You just made a choice that is going to get you to that goal more quickly. When you reach that lower body fat percentage, your body is going to be operating more efficiently, your metabolism rate is going to be higher, and you will be able to burn fat more quickly than you can right now. Once you have reached that point, you will be able to enjoy your favorite dessert without sabotaging your goals.

The bottom line is this. Discover what your underlying motivation is.

Write it down. Stay focused on it every day and use it as a force to aid you in making good choices on a daily basis to achieve the goals and dreams you have for your body and your life.

Goal Setting

Goal setting is extremely important because it gives you a means of monitoring how and when you have achieved success. What are your goals? What is it that you really want to achieve with your body and your life? If you don't have goals you won't know exactly what you are working to achieve. Goals will help keep you focused, and the baby steps that you make towards fulfilling them will keep you motivated. Now that you know what your motivation is, sit down and write out exactly what it is that you are going to accomplish throughout your transformation period.

To help you, develop **SMART** goals based on the following criteria:

Specific so that it is easy to discern what the goal entails;

Measurable by numeric amounts;

Action-oriented with a plan for how to achieve them;

Realistic so that you are not setting yourself up for failure;

Time-bound with a specific date in the future by which they will be attained.

When embarking on a personal and physical transformation, it is easy to be overzealous when outlining your goals. Please pay special attention to the "R" in SMART and be sure to set goals that they are realistic for you to achieve. It is better to set a realistic goal and achieve it than to set an unrealistic goal and experience frustration from not being able to accomplish it.

For example, if you need to lose 50 pounds, please don't make it your goal to lose that within one month. This is an unrealistic goal because it would not be healthy to lose that much weight in such a short period of time, and it would be extremely difficult to do so by using safe and effective methods. A better goal would be to lose 10 pounds in a month.

There are two different types of goals, long-term or life goals and short-term goals. Long-term or life goals are things that you would like to accomplish over the next five years or possibly throughout the rest of your life. These could be anything from achieving a higher level of education, starting a family, buying a home, saving retirement funds, being financially independent or achieving complete mental and emotional wellness.

Keeping in mind the criteria of a SMART goal, take a moment now to write down what your major long-term goals are within all facets of your life.

Next up are the short-term goals. These can be anything you want to accomplish within the next week, month, year or five years. This could be attaining a promotion at work, losing a specific amount of body fat, making changes to your current nutrition habits or getting more active in a community or physical activity group. Take a moment now and write out your short-term goals using the SMART goal criteria. For example, if you goal is to lose weight, please be particular on how much weight you are going to lose and by what date you will have achieved this goal.

Once your goals are written out, you need a plan of action. It's great to have goals and things that you want in life, but honestly, if you don't take ACTION towards those goals, they are never going to come to fruition. We need to know how you are going to accomplish each of these aspirations. Next to each goal write down the steps you must take in order for it to become a reality. Going back to our weight loss example, if your goal is to lose 10 pounds over the next month your plan of action might be to sign up for a gym membership (if you don't already have one), stop specific negative habits that are setting you back (such as eating chocolate or ice cream at 11 p.m.), commit to at least four to five cardio sessions into your weekly routine and at least two to three strength training sessions, start eating a healthy breakfast and drink water consistently throughout the day.

The bottom line is this, in order to achieve a transformation you must have goals you are working toward. Set long term and short term goals for yourself. Develop a plan of action on how to achieve them, and start working towards making those goals a reality in your life today!

The Keys to a Healthy Relationship

Healthy relationships are crucial keys to overall happiness, especially when we are talking about the relationship with your spouse or significant other, but what makes up a healthy relationship? Now trust me, we have both been in bad relationships, in negative and unhealthy relationships, and sometimes it does take going through these to truly know what you want and need in a partner for life. You can learn a lot about yourself even through bad relationships, but long term, if you want true happiness in life, you have to have a partner that you love and are happy to be with every single day.

Our relationship is quite unique. We live together, we work together, we train together, and we are together 24 hours a day. For many couples that may not work. But for us, that is how we like it and wouldn't have it any other way. We have learned a lot about each other, and have learned how to compromise on the small stuff (Micah gets to play video games as long as Diana gets to watch The Bachelor and Biggest Loser). We have learned when to give each other space, and when it is important to drop all that we are doing to pay attention to what the other is saying. We are best friends. We have similar goals and aspirations. Our trust level and confidence in our love for one another is 100% (which is crucial especially in the business that we work), and most importantly, our faith is the same. We have discovered that we are both Time people, meaning that the way that we best express love is by giving our time to each other and to the people important in our lives. The way we best understand love is by people giving of their time to us. This is why being together so much works for us and our relationship.

We've found that the top points to be connected on for a relationship to work are: Spiritual, emotional, physical, financial and life goals. If any of these areas is out of balance, the relationship will likely be off balance as well. Let's look a little deeper at each of these areas and see if there are areas that you and your loved one can work on together. If you're single, this is good to know as you look for a future mate!

1) **Emotional** - This means having a like-minded connection, having a bond with your partner that allows you to know what they are feeling or thinking without them even saying a word. It means being best friends with your partner and knowing what you need to give of yourself emotionally for them to be satisfied, while receiving from them what you need in order to feel loved. Confidence is a big piece of the puzzle when it comes to the emotional connection. The healthiest and most loving relationships are the ones where both partners trust each other implicitly and are secure in the commitment their partner has made to them. When you are on the same level emotionally as your partner, you could be with that person 24/7 and still want more.

2) **Physical-** Physical attraction has to be part of the equation at some level. You may hear that men are more focused on looks and women say they aren't that important, but honestly a physical connection and chemistry is very important for a healthy relationship. Looks certainly aren't everything. They can be taken away in an instant and they will fade with time. What is important is that, in your personal opinion, the person you are in a relationship with is beautiful and attractive to YOU. Wouldn't you want to wake up to the person you love everyday and think to yourself, "Wow I'm the luckiest person in the world. Not only are they great inside but they are also beautiful on the outside (in your mind)." It is important to take care of yourself physically for your partner and vice versa, your partner should take care of themselves for you. A partner who works out, makes healthy eating choices, takes care of their body not just for themselves, but also for you, to keep that attraction alive... that's HOT.

3) **Spiritual-** Having a connection spiritually is another crucial piece of the puzzle. It is important to have a partner who thinks like you in matters of faith, spirituality and how life should be lived. If you and your spouse have conflicting views on the right and wrong ways to live life or differing religious perspectives, that is a warning sign for trouble down the road.

If you have differing opinions on what a positive and productive lifestyle consists of you should be aware. If you have a partner that wants to go out to clubs all the time and get wasted but you would rather spend time doing more productive and positive activities, you must be prepared for friction to build. If you want to go to church on a regular basis, but you have a partner that doesn't believe the same as you and has no interest or desire to go to church, down the road this is going to cause friction. Finding a partner with similar spiritual and lifestyle views is important to a happy and positive relationship.

4) **Financial**- When it comes to being financially compatible with your significant other it doesn't mean that you both have to be rich or poor. It does mean that you have open communication about where you are financially and how monetary issues will be handled in the future. Satisfaction and happiness are attainable in a relationship regardless of how much money flows into the home, but a relationship works best when both partners are passionate about what they do for a living.

5) **Life Goals** – Another important factor and key to a healthy relationship is having similar life goals. Probably the best example of this is if you want to have several children and you are in a relationship with someone who doesn't want children at all, or vice versa. Perhaps you are someone who truly wants to get married, and you are dating someone who says that they never want to marry. These are big issues that you should discuss with your mate in the early stages of your relationship.

It may not seem important in those first few months of dating someone, and maybe they are issues you feel you would be able to change their mind on in the future. But chances are, they won't change their mind, and long term, these can be heart-breaking deal breakers. Discuss with your significant other what their long-term vision is for their life, for their career, and for your future together. You don't have to have the exact same life goals as your mate, but be sure that the two of you are going to both be happy with whatever compromises have to be made.

If you aren't compatible with your companion in one or more of these areas, tension and insecurities may build up over time that can eventually break up the relationship. You can't change people. Sometimes, if someone is looking to better themselves, you can be patient and do your best to guide them to a more efficient lifestyle, but ultimately it's their choice. Honestly, if you are pushy about trying to change your partner when they aren't ready for it, they may become resentful and actually do the opposite of what you are hoping!

If you are married and find that you are incompatible in some of these areas, then it would be wise to seek counseling in order to find those compromises that will help you and your spouse work through things and create a happier, healthier future together. If you are dating someone who you aren't compatible with in these areas, you may need to reconsider the relationship and possibly let it go and move on. You deserve a healthy, happy and positive relationship. Don't settle for someone who is not right for you. That right person will come along and when they do GO FOR IT!

So, now that we have talked about motivational factors, goal setting and healthy relationships, let's take a closer look at Hitch Fit, and what transformation is really about.

What is Transformation Training?

As you may have noticed, here in Hitch Fit world we love to use the word transformation. In the dictionary, the best fitting definition of transformation is this, "*A marked change, as in appearance or character, usually for the better.*" We love that the dictionary even indicates that a transformation isn't just about what happens to you on the outside with your physical appearance, but it also entails an inner change. A change in character, or a change in the way you see yourself, in turn changes how others see you. A true transformation can change your course in life, your career, relationships, and your beliefs about yourself and the world around you.

The programs that we put together for clients, whether we get the chance to work with them in person, or online, are focused on the most efficient and effective transformation possible.

In today's society there is a lot out there that says that if you just make small changes on a daily basis, that you will lose weight and be healthier. If you just cut out the soda, or if you just take the stairs or park farther away from work, you can reap some health benefits. Is this true? Yes of course. And if you are still in a state of mind of not wanting to take full responsibility for all of your choices and undergo a complete transformation, then something is certainly better than nothing.

There's nothing wrong with taking small, slow baby steps. We hold nothing against people who take that route, it is just important to understand that if that is the amount of work and effort you are willing to put in, then your results and the outcome of that effort will be small and slow as well. Making small, progressive, slow changes to your eating and exercise habits will absolutely get you on the path to success, but it may take years depending on how de-conditioned or over fat you are currently. The key word here is progressive. If you commit to walking five minutes a day, but never progress to ten minutes…twenty minutes...thirty minutes, then your body may initially make some changes, but then it will adapt and you will hit a plateau.

There are a lot of people out there looking for big outcomes, big results, but with little effort and little change. The point blank truth is this, if you're looking for big outcomes, then little changes aren't going to get you there. If you're ready to make some big changes and major commitments, then you CAN get to where you want to be in a much more time efficient and effective manner.

When we talk about transformation training, we are talking about asking you to commit to making big changes in your life. Remember, you are absolutely capable of taking full responsibility of your actions immediately. Thinking that you need a transition period or that you need to slowly adapt is just a mental road block that you have set up for yourself. Transforming your lifestyle means that you are committing to tossing out the old and adopting the new, giving yourself a fresh and healthy start, embarking on a new fit and healthy lifestyle with no plans of ever going back to your old ways.

Transformation training means that you are making a commitment, not just to us, but to yourself, that you are ready and willing to get yourself to a place where you are able to function on your highest level as a human being.

Now we don't encourage unhealthy weight loss by any means. We encourage our clients to set reasonable goals for the time limits that they have available. We will never tell someone that they should come in and plan on shedding 100 pounds in 12 weeks, that would be unsafe and unhealthy, but we do promote that you can shed 25-30 pounds and in some cases more than that, in a 12 week time period with proper nutrition and training. If you've got 40-50 pounds to lose, then you can achieve that in a 16 week period of time. If it's higher than that, then your transformation journey is going to take longer, which is ok, as long as you are prepared to stay focused and give yourself the best possible chance of getting to that goal, in a healthy way, as quickly as possible.

We ask a lot of our clients. We don't believe in starvation diets. We do believe in keeping our clients fed and having them work and train hard in order to achieve their goals. Ultimately this combination of proper nutrition and training serves to not just transform them visually, but also makes them stronger than they have ever been physically. Having that physical strength makes them stronger mentally than they have ever been as well.

Transformation training means that you are giving 100% effort. Everyone's 100% is going to be a little bit different. Some people are already in good condition and working towards getting in great condition. Some people have never stepped foot into a gym or lifted a weight or walked on a treadmill in their life. Their 100% is of course going to be quite different. We don't care. We don't care if your 100% is doing 5 minutes of walking, if that's all you've got, then that's what we expect you to give.

On the nutrition side of things, during transformation the more 100% that you are with your eating, the more quickly you are going to get to your goals. A transformation phase does not last forever. You're not giving up your favorite cheats and treats for a lifetime. When you have achieved your goals there are healthy ways to incorporate treats back into a balanced style of eating. For some, being spot on with nutrition comes as a greater challenge, especially with crazy work schedules, frequent travel, or kids and spouses at home who aren't following the same nutritional guidelines. Even with these obstacles, if you truly want to achieve your goals, you have to believe in yourself and your ability to make the best choices on every occasion.

Transformation will be progressive. It will be tough, and it will push you beyond the limits that you thought possible for yourself. The goal of transformation is to get you to where you want to be. The work is going to be hard to get there, and it's going to take discipline and consistency, and YES you do have what it takes! We ask you to work very hard to get to where you want to be, and then once you've hit that golden mark, whatever it may be for you, you will be ready for the next phase, maintenance.

You achieve your transformation, now what?

You've busted your booty, you've been perfect with your nutrition and you have it, the physique that you always hoped and dreamed you would have! It's a wonderful feeling. But now that you have it, what's the next step? Do you have to continue to perform transformation training in order to maintain your results? Does your eating still have to stay as strict?

The answer is no. Maintenance periods are wonderful because now you get to reap the benefits of your hard work. You will be able to increase your calorie intake per day by around 300-500 calories typically, and that will allow your body to stay within a good healthy range at all times.

This does NOT mean that you get to go back to how you were eating before, and it does not mean that you get to stop working out or quit going to the gym. If you go back to your old eating habits, or if you stop working out altogether, guess what? Your body is going to start going back to exactly what it looked like before.

Hitch Fit is a lifestyle. It's a consistent way of living, day in and day out, for the rest of your life. The nutrition programs that we put together are blueprints for how you should be eating for the rest of your life. The staples of a healthy diet (which we will go over in an upcoming chapter) are the same for the rest of your life. There is never a time that you will be able to go back to eating fast food on a regular basis, eating loads of sugar and sweets, skipping breakfast and then binging later in the day, unless you are planning on getting your old unfit body back.

In general, your cardio workouts should still be about 3-4 days per week for anywhere from 20-45 minutes. If you were obese to begin with, then your maintenance cardio levels may always have to be a bit higher than this, if you were leaner to begin with, you may be able to maintain your body fat with fewer cardio sessions per week. (For example, Diana's off season cardio consists of 2-3 days of 20-25 minutes of cardio).

Strength training always needs to be a part of your lifestyle as well, if you stop training you will feel "soft and squishy", your muscles will atrophy and shrink, and your metabolism will slow down. Strength train a minimum of twice per week, and anywhere up to 6 days per week (on training split routines). Vary your workouts on a regular basis. Don't get stuck in the rut of doing the same routine over and over again or your body will stop responding to it.

It does make a difference what your starting body fat and weight were as you start your transition into maintenance. If you have lost a large amount of weight and were either overweight, obese or morbidly obese in the beginning phases, then you will have to be more careful with your eating for the rest of your life. One of the reasons is because when your body becomes over fat, it produces more and more fat cells to store all of the excess you have been feeding it. When you lose weight, the fat cells do not go away, they simply shrink. However, the number of them is always going to be higher (unless you are considering having skin removal surgery or something similar, which is only advised in extreme cases). This means your body has created a physical environment that is much more prone to filling those fat cells back up.

The key to maintaining your body is by finding a healthy balance. A good rule of thumb is to eat clean and stay on track at least 80% of the time when you are trying to maintain your body. For the most part, you are going to eat the same, 5 to 6 small meals per day, with healthy combinations of fat, carbohydrates and protein. You will satisfy yourself with plenty of lean meats, vegetables and fruit, as well as healthy fat sources and whole grain carbohydrates. But you will also have some room for cheats and treats!

You will also be able to add in more of the foods that are healthy for you, but not the best for transformation purposes including items such as low fat or skim dairy products, a little more fruit, and a wider variety of additions to your meals like cheese and salsa. Moderation is ALWAYS the key though.

If you go by the 80% rule, let's say that you are eating 6 meals per day for a total of 42 meals per week. That means that at least 33-34 of your meals during that time period will be clean and on point, but you have room for some small cheats at 6 or 7 meals during that period of time. That DOES NOT mean that you have room to eat 6 or 7 buckets of ice cream. Even your cheats should be in moderation. You have to remember that your body can only handle so many calories at a time, and even though your metabolism will be faster when you are leaner and more fit, if you over consume too many calories all at once, your body will have no choice but to store those as fat weight!

During a maintenance phase, it's wise to keep an eye on your weight and body fat. You should always stay within a couple pound range of what your ideal weight is. If the scale starts going progressively up, you will know that you are overdoing it and need to reign things back in. Clean up your diet and increase your cardio levels until you are back to where you want to be, and then you can go back to the maintenance rules.

CHAPTER TEN
NUTRITION

Nutrition. You hear this word tossed around in the health and fitness industry all the time. You hear that you are supposed to eat "right," but what does that really mean? It's so confusing with all of the weight loss gimmicks, misguided advertising and marketing schemes that are out there. We are going to be real with you and break this down in the simplest way possible to get you headed in the right direction to properly nourish your body and achieve your physical transformation.

This is one of our favorite quotes. On average, we say this to people 2 to 3 times per day: "Abs are NOT made in the gym. They are made in the kitchen." This statement is absolutely true and pertains not just to being able to see a "six pack" set of abs but also to any other physical fitness goal that you might have such as leaner legs, glutes, arms, hips, etc. The desire to have any one of these is only doable if you are willing to spend some time in the kitchen as well as the gym.

This is an education process for you. We don't want you to eat certain foods just because we said so. We want you to know WHY you are eating them and what they are going to do for you. There is no single diet plan that works for EVERY body. Figuring out how to lose weight is a matter of figuring out YOUR body. What works for us or the fit guy or girl at the gym that you admire and aspire to look like may not work for you. You have to figure out what works for YOU. The diet plan for a 64-year-old man is going to be completely different than the plan for a 24-year-old female because their bodies simply don't function in the same way. Losing weight and shedding body fat boils down to a couple of factors which we will go over now.

First is calorie consumption versus calorie expenditure. A calorie is simply a unit of energy. If you are consuming more energy than your body is utilizing to function in a day, then that energy has to be stored somewhere. If it isn't used right away, it can either be stored in muscles as glycogen to be used at a later time for energy, or it stores as fat. Bottom line is in order to lose weight and shed body fat you have to be consuming less than you are expending in a day.

Sounds easy right? Well, not really. If it were JUST about calories in versus calories out, then starvation diets would be an effective way to get lean, or you could just eat Twinkies® all day and get lean, or you could not eat all day and eat all your caloric intake for the day in the evening, and get lean. We hear over and over again from people with these types of habits, that they don't understand why they are still GAINING weight, even when they are not eating above their calorie recommendations for the day.

Here's the thing. Your body is smart, and it can only utilize a certain amount of fuel at a time. Overloading your system with a massive calorie consumption in one sitting is like trying to pour 20 gallons of fuel into a 10 gallon tank, and then wondering why it's all spilling out. Your body also can tell when it is starving. When you go for long periods of time without eating, you are sending signals to your body that you will not be feeding it for quite some time. Your body will respond by sending an alert to all systems to SLOW down and preserve as much energy as possible. It also encourages your body to store fat because during this time of famine, the most important thing is that your body survives!

Your metabolism, the rate at which your body burns off calories in order to sustain itself, is slowed down significantly when you are starving yourself and not getting sufficient calories. That makes it even slower at processing food as energy. This, in turn, contributes to the continuous vicious cycle of fat gain, even IF your calorie consumption isn't over what your daily caloric intake should be.

*The lesson to learn here is that you DO have to be in a calorie deficit in order to lose body fat. If you consume over what you are expending in a day, it will store as fat. This overspill simply has no place else to go! But the other rule to remember is that your body can only utilize a small amount of calories at a time, so eating all your calories at once or starving your body throughout the day and only eating 1 or 2 times daily, will be counterproductive to shedding body fat and getting lean!

The type of calories you are consuming is equally important. There are foods that will promote fat gain regardless of if you go over your caloric needs. If you think that fat loss is as simple as a matter of calories in versus calories out, then you ought to be able to eat candy, cookies and Twinkies® all day as long as you are eating fewer calories than your body is expending. Wouldn't that make sense and be true? Let's take a closer look.

FOOD CLASSIFICATION

Foods are classified into different categories: carbohydrates, protein and fats. We will take a look at these food types in more depth in an upcoming chapter, but for now, just know that these are the basics. Many junk foods such as cookies, chips, soda and pastries are classified as simple carbohydrates. They are typically loaded with sugar. Though all carbohydrates, even the healthy complex ones, break down into your body as sugar, the digestion rate for these simple sugar foods is much faster. When you consume carbohydrates, whether simple or complex, they break down into a simple sugar called glucose and are absorbed into your blood stream.

Your body can only handle so much sugar in the blood at one time. It is constantly in a state of trying to keep blood glucose levels stable. When you eat a high-sugar junk food that converts very quickly into blood sugar, your blood glucose levels will sky rocket quickly. To get back to balance, your body will release a hormone called insulin. The purpose of insulin is to find someplace to store this extra sugar so that it doesn't stay in the blood for long periods of time. When the insulin levels rise, the sugar is quickly exported from the blood. If there is no room for this sugar to be stored in muscle tissue or the liver, then it will store as fat. The more frequently throughout the day that you eat these types of foods, the more frequently your insulin levels are going to spike and your body will go into fat-storing mode.

The bigger the meal is, or the more junk you eat in one sitting, the more insulin your body is going to have to produce to rid the blood of all that glucose. In an unfit person especially, the majority of these calories will store as fat. Those who have had poor eating habits for long periods of time, are overweight or obese and don't exercise actually can be at an even greater disadvantage. The constant spikes of insulin can make your muscles resistant to taking it in and storing it as glycogen for later use. Therefore, any spikes in insulin can easily transport that sugar to fat cells, so the fat can easily and readily continue to grow fatter. This is one example of how you can continue to gain fat weight even if you under eat your calories.

High fat foods such as fast food and fried food will lead to significant weight and fat gain easily. The reason is because fat, gram for gram, is the most calorically dense nutrient. Carbohydrates are 4 calories per gram, as is protein. Fat is 9 calories per gram, so the calories will add up quickly and it is very easy to over consume what your daily calories should be for the day. Now this doesn't mean eliminate fats from your diet altogether. There are healthy fats (which we go over in a separate section), that are beneficial for your health and for your fitness goals. It is just important to understand that all fats are not created equal.

If you consistently eat foods high in saturated fat, this fat goes into your blood stream clogging it up, and forcing your heart to push harder to get the blood moving through your body. This undue stress on your heart can lead to many unwanted health complications including heart attack and stroke.

The reason WHY we have our clients eat the way they do, and WHY we recommend the foods that we do in this book is because they have the **reverse** effect. The foods that we recommend are intended to keep your blood sugar levels even and stable, thus promoting low insulin levels and production of the opposite hormone glucagon, which helps to free fat from storage in your body.

The foods that we recommend are slow digesting. They have a higher thermogenic effect, meaning the act of just eating them is burning more calories. They are the foods that are best for aiding in the maintenance and development of lean muscle tissue, which will in turn speed up your metabolism and help your body to become a fat burning machine. They are the foods that will get your body to your goals in the most efficient and effective way possible. The moral of the story here is that it isn't just about calories in versus calories out. The type of foods that you choose is also an extremely important factor if your goal is to achieve a lean and fit physique!

Timing of your calories is another important piece of the puzzle which we touched upon earlier. We encourage our clients to eat small meals frequently throughout the day, and there is a reason for that. Your body can only process so many calories at one time. If you eat small meals of the right types of foods throughout the day, then your body will be able to fully utilize those calories for fuel. It will also help to keep your blood insulin levels in check all day long, and it will keep your energy levels balanced throughout the entire day.

***Another important point is that under-eating can be just as detrimental to your health as overeating. This is one of the reasons why we detest the fad diets. Your body is burning calories ALL the time, whether you are sitting, standing, eating, sleeping, breathing or exercising intensely. Your body is burning calories at all times. It takes energy for your body to function even when you are completely still. The amount of calories that your body burns during the day if you sat perfectly still and didn't move at all is called your BMR or Basal Metabolic Rate. If you go on a crash diet and starve yourself by consuming less calories than your body needs to function, then your body thinks that it is starving. It slows down your BMR even more, trying to preserve calories as much as possible. If there aren't sufficient calories to use as fuel, your body will also turn to lean muscle tissue and use THAT as fuel, so your lean mass would decrease, and this again drops the BMR. When people go on starvation diets, they end up losing muscle and slowing their body way down. Then when they go off the diet and go back to old eating habits where the calorie intake goes up, their body is slower, less able to burn calories up for fuel, and more likely to store these added calories as fat.

HOW MANY CALORIES SHOULD YOU BE EATING IN A DAY?

This is one of the things that we help each client out with via the Hitch Fit Online Training Program. To be perfectly honest, there is no exact answer to this question. The amount of calories that we actually burn in a day varies every single day. If you had to park the car further than normal at work or the grocery store, or if you ended up running more errands than expected, or if you were sick one day and ended up having to stay home in bed, each of these days your actual calorie burn is going to be different. However, even though there is no 100% accurate way, there are ways that we can get very good estimations of the range that you should be in to appropriately achieve your goals. One easy method to determine minimum calorie intake per day is by first figuring out your body fat percentage. Fat is not metabolically active. You don't need to feed fat. Muscle on the other hand is very metabolically active, and you want to feed it so that you maintain it, or increase it. Let's say that you are a 220 pound man and your body fat is at 25%. When you multiply your weight times your body fat, you will find that you have 55 pounds of fat on your body. The rest we refer to as Lean Body Mass - that means all the muscle, tissue, organs, bones, and everything else on you that IS NOT fat. When you subtract fat weight from lean body mass 220-55 you get 165 lbs. Take this lean body mass number and multiply by 10 in order to get a rough estimate of the very bare minimum of calories that you should eat in the day in order to allow your body to properly function. For this person that very bare minimum number is 1650, so they should never drop below that 1650 calories per day. Now this is the base metabolic rate, which means that daily activity and exercise aren't being factored into the equation. When this client is put on a progressive workout program, the calories eaten per day will be quite a bit higher and will still allow him to be in a caloric deficit and burn off body fat, without starving.

***Other factors that we take into account when putting together nutrition programs for our clients are age, whether you are male or female, what your body type is (more on this in a later chapter), what your daily activity level is (do you have an active job or a sedentary job), and of course body fat which we mentioned above. We ask all of our clients to provide us with this information in the beginning of their programs. The reason is because it gives us the best picture, and the best way of determining where your caloric intake for the day should be in order to be most successful on your program.

In very broad and general terms, the majority of females are going to be eating somewhere in the 1200-1800 calorie range per day for fat loss, and males are going to be eating in the 2000 – 2600 calorie range depending on all the factors listed above.

WHAT IF YOUR GOAL IS TO GAIN MUSCLE?

While we are still on the topic of nutrition, let's shift gears for a moment and talk about those of you who are coming to Hitch Fit not because you want to lose weight or fat, but because you want to gain muscle and build size. In order to gain a significant amount of muscle, your caloric intake needs to be higher than what your calorie burn is for the day. Instead of putting your body in a caloric deficit, it needs to be in a caloric surplus. It can be just as challenging to put on size as it is to lose body fat, especially if you are someone who leads a busy lifestyle and often skips meals and loses out on valuable calories. You have to EAT to build muscle. During a true muscle building phase, you will not be leaning down (even though a lot of magazines will tell you that you can get huge muscles and get shredded at the same time, the fact of the matter is these are two different phases and require two different training and eating strategies).

You CAN put on some muscle in the initial phases of a leaning program, that is common especially in beginners. However, you will not put on a lot of muscle during leaning. Vice versa, if you eat the larger amount of calories from clean and healthy foods, you will gain mostly muscle but may still put on some fat weight. This can be monitored if you keep a close eye on how your weight and body fat are rising. If weight is going up quickly, but muscle isn't going up too much, that means you are overeating and gaining more fat than muscle. If your weight is not going up at all that means you are not eating enough to gain size. If your weight is going up gradually and body fat is not going up significantly, that means that you are doing what you need to do! If you eat a lot of junk food while you are building and bulking, your chances of gaining higher amounts of fat weight and less muscle are greatly increased.

We recommend that if you are thinking of building and bulking, that you actually go through a leaning out process first. The reason is, because when you are leaner you will better be able to see what areas of your body need the most improvement and growth. The second reason is because if your body fat is higher, and you are bulking and eating higher calories, your body is far more likely to put on more fat weight through the process than if you are leaner at the start.

(***Most of you reading this book are doing so because you are already a current Hitch Fit client, whether online or in person. If you are not a client and would like more information on the programs we have to offer please visit our website www.hitchfit.com. We put the whole program together for each of our clients and take the guesswork out of the equation. We offer Lose Weight/Feel Great programs, Fitness Model and Bikini Model Programs, Muscle Building, Couples and Bridal Programs, Post Pregnancy Programs, and full Figure and Fitness Model competitor Prep programs.)

There are three major food categories that are essential to your diet and to your overall health which we mentioned earlier. Let's take a look at these categories in a bit more depth. They include protein, carbohydrates and fats, and eating them in the proper combinations will aid you in transforming your body into the fit physique you desire.

PROTEIN

What is protein, and why do our bodies need it? Protein is the main building block for your fit and healthy body. There are a lot of great benefits to eating protein. We already know that it aids in muscle building, repairs body tissue and preserves lean muscle tissue. Protein also aids in immune function and aids in body fat loss as it stimulates the metabolism. Protein will keep you feeling full and will help you to overcome any cravings to make unhealthy food choices. In my opinion, protein is the most important nutrient in your body for the simple fact that it is found literally everywhere in your body, nails, skin, blood, muscle tissue and internal organs.

Protein is made up of amino acids, which are essential to the human body. They aid in the development of muscle and muscle growth and repair. They are responsible for all of the body's enzymes and also play a key role in sleep, normalizing moods, concentration and attention.

When you eat protein, your stomach and small intestines break it down into amino acids, which can then be utilized for all of these functions. If you don't consume enough protein, your body will not be able to build or maintain lean muscle mass. In fact, you will actually lose precious muscle tissue because your body will have to use it for fuel. The reason you don't want this to happen is because your metabolism will slow down and your body will not be as efficient at burning fat.

In order to achieve a lean physique, your body must be burning fat and not muscle. To ensure that you consume enough protein, a good rule of thumb is to ingest 1 to 2 grams of protein per pound of body weight per day. If you are looking to maintain the muscle you currently have and burn off fat, you will want to stick to about 1 gram per pound. If your goal is to gain additional muscle mass you will want to increase that amount and consume around 1.5 to 2 grams per pound of bodyweight. There is no need to eat more than the recommended amounts of protein. If you consume more than your body can utilize, it will go to waste and will be excreted.

To determine the amount of protein that you need to intake per meal, simply multiply your bodyweight by the grams per pound you should be consuming based on your fitness goals. Divide that number by the amount of meals that you will be eating in a day, which should be anywhere from 4 to 7, and that is the amount of protein grams you should be consuming per meal.

For most people, that amount is going to be 20 to 35 grams of protein per meal. For example, a 135-pound woman who wants to lose body fat and maintain muscle mass will consume 1 gram of protein per pound. She will be eating five meals per day so that means she needs to consume 27 grams of protein at each of those meals, preferably from a complete protein source. Be sure you read labels in order to determine your portion sizes.

There are two types of proteins: complete and incomplete. Complete proteins are found in most products of animal origin, such as meat, poultry, eggs, cheese, fish and milk. They are called "complete" because they contain all of the amino acids, that are essential to your body.

There are nine essential amino acids (histidine, isoleucine, leucine, valine, lysine, methionine, phenylalanine, threonine and tryptophan) and 11 non-essential amino acids (alanine, arginine, asparagines, aspartic acid, cysteine, glutamic acid, glutamine, glycine, praline, serine and tyrosine). The essential amino acids must be provided to your body from your diet. The non-essentials can be created by your body so they aren't considered essential. Complete proteins should be consumed at every single meal.

Here is a list of food sources that will provide your body with protein:

• Boneless, skinless chicken breast

• Skinless turkey breast or lean ground turkey

• Egg whites

• Lean ground meats (chicken, turkey, lamb, beef)

• Lean cuts of meat (beef (filet), lamb, veal)

• Game meats (venison, bison, rabbit)

• Low-fat or non-fat dairy products, such as yogurt, cottage cheese, or milk

• Fish (tuna, salmon, mahi-mahi, orange roughy, haddock, pollock, snapper, trout, tuna, swordfish, mackerel, halibut, sea bass, catfish, cod, flounder, etc.)

• Shellfish (shrimp, clams, crab, lobster, squid (calamari), crayfish, mussels, octopus, etc.)

• Soybean products (tofu, textured vegetable protein (TVP), soy bean curd, etc.)

• Bean Burgers (Veggie Burgers, Garden Burgers)

• Protein powder substitute (whey and casein)

Vegetables and beans are examples of incomplete proteins because on their own they are lacking some of the essential amino acids. However, it is possible to create a complete protein by combining two foods together, for example, when you eat beans and rice or rice cakes and peanut butter.

Most of the protein grams should come from complete protein sources. The best sources to choose are egg whites, chicken, turkey, white fish, tuna, salmon and whey or casein protein powder. Red meat is not easily digestible. If you choose to eat it on occasion, choose a leaner cut of meat such as a filet.

Dairy is an important component to your diet overall because it plays a part in protecting our bodies from injury and disease. It provides our bodies with the vital nutrients calcium and vitamin D. If you don't get enough of these, you will have a higher risk of developing osteoporosis. Though dairy is essential to your diet in its whole forms, it is very high in fat and calories, which is why you need to choose the fat-free or low-fat versions and consume them in moderation. Dairy should be a regular staple of your diet during maintenance periods, however during transformation it is not the best protein choice to get you to your goals. We prefer that dairy is limited or eliminated during transformation period, and incorporated back in during maintenance. Since it is a great source of calcium and vitamin D, please be sure to supplement with these two, or find a multi vitamin that is enriched with them as well. This is also the case if you are lactose intolerant and can't eat dairy at all.

One great way to make sure you are getting the right amount of protein into your diet is by drinking protein shakes. It is absolutely possible to attain your daily requirements for protein from natural food sources, however it can be very time consuming to prepare all of that food. Shakes are especially convenient for the hectic and busy lifestyles we all lead.

We recommend you find a whey protein isolate powder. *Read the label and make sure that protein isolate is the first ingredient listed.* Whey concentrate is a lower quality of protein and doesn't digest or absorb as effectively. Therefore, you aren't going to get the most bang for your buck if you purchase a whey protein concentrate instead of an isolate.

Casein protein is a slow-digesting, high-source protein. It feeds your muscles over a longer period of time than whey protein. The best times to use casein are in the morning and at night before you go to bed.

An optimum shake would be made with a combination of whey protein isolate and casein. This is the ideal blend for promoting the growth of lean muscle tissue. Make your shake by mixing your protein powder with water or skim milk in a blender.

For those who don't consume animal products, soy protein is a suitable alternative. Just as with whey protein, you want to find a soy product that has soy protein isolate as the main ingredient.

The most important thing to remember about protein is to consume the adequate amount of protein for your fitness goals at every meal because it will help you develop, retain and increase lean muscle tissue, which in turn increases your metabolism, allowing your body to be a fat-burning machine.

Carbohydrates

With all the hype about low-carb and no-carb diets over the past couple of years, you (like millions of people) may believe carbohydrates are evil. We assure you that your body NEEDS carbohydrates in order to properly function. They are crucial to developing a complete nutrition plan. Carbohydrates are the preferred source of energy for your body. Without them your body can't function efficiently and effectively.

Carbs are what give us the energy to train hard, and the right types of carbs will keep you full and satisfied. They supply us with vitamins, minerals and fiber, and can be stored in our muscles and liver and utilized later for energy. They are needed for the central nervous system, kidneys, brain and muscles to function properly.

But wait! Before you head to the pantry to have a little carb indulgence, keep reading. There is some truth behind all the anti-carb hype. If you are eating the wrong type of carbs, eating them at the wrong times or eating them in higher portions than your body can utilize, they will in fact be stored very quickly in your body as fat.

Diets that completely eliminate carbohydrates are not going to be beneficial for you in the long term. The weight that you lose on a no carb or super low carb diet is mainly going to be water weight and precious lean muscle tissue. When your body is deprived of carbs, it resorts to using muscle and protein as its energy source. Essentially, your metabolism slows down and lean body mass decreases. The majority of people who have lost tons of "weight" on diets like the old Atkins plan mostly gained all their weight back and then some as soon as they caved to carb cravings, incorporated carbs back into their diets or reverted back to their old eating habits.

There are two types of carbohydrates: complex and simple. Complex carbs break down over a longer period of time and therefore, sustain us for longer periods of time. They come in two subgroups: starchy and fibrous. These are known as the "healthy carbohydrates." When you are trying to get lean, the majority of your carbohydrates will come from this group.

Starchy carbs include rice, grains, potatoes, pasta and wholegrain bread. Fibrous carbs include asparagus, cauliflower, broccoli, onions and spinach and add volume to your meals without a lot of extra calories. They also contain lots of vitamins and minerals and should be incorporated into every diet.

Simple carbohydrates are simple sugars, and they don't have the nutritional value of the complex carbohydrates. Sugar comes in a variety of forms, including milk, honey, chocolate, cakes, etc. This form of carbohydrate will more readily store as fat in your body. Simple carbs will spike your insulin levels which will cause them to be stored as fat. Fruits are simple sugars, but they are a healthier option and do have nutritional value due to fiber content, vitamins and minerals. The best choices for fruits are apples, raspberries, strawberries, melons and oranges. The amount of these should still be minimal, and a good diet is going to include more vegetables than fruits.

It is important to choose the right type of carbohydrates on your path towards a lean physique. The right types of carbs are going to aid you in your fat loss quest whereas the wrong ones are going to set you back and cause you to gain unwanted weight. Foods such as cookies, cakes, sodas and other sweets are high in simple carbohydrates and sugar and will store as fat. Foods such as chips, French fries, bagels, white breads and pastas are high in carbs, and will also store as fat very easily. Avoid the non nutritional carbs, stick with healthy carbs, and your body will be energized and will become a fat-burning machine.

Carbs are found in a wide variety of foods. Here is a list of the foods from which you should derive your carbohydrates:

- Fibrous Carbs: This category encompasses all your vegetables including broccoli, Brussel sprouts, squash, spinach, tomatoes, zucchini, green beans, cauliflower, green or white asparagus, artichokes, lettuce, green/red/orange/yellow peppers, bamboo shoots, sprouts, red and green cabbage, eggplant, collard greens, onions, kale, okra, leeks, cucumbers, mushrooms, celery and swiss chard.

Next up are the starchy carbs. There are natural starchy carbs that haven't been processed in any way, and those are going to be your best choice for this category. They include:

- Sweet potatoes or yams;

- Beans (chick peas, black beans, black eyed peas, soy beans, butter beans, split peas, white beans, lima beans, pinto beans, navy beans, garbanzo beans, kidney beans, etc.);

- Potatoes (Red and White);

- Peas;

- Brown rice;

- Corn;

- Rye;

- Other root vegetables (turnips, carrots, beets, radishes);

- Oatmeal, Cream of Wheat, Cream of Rice, Cream of Rye;

- Rye; and

- Millet.

The next group are also starchy carbohydrates. They are not all-natural and have gone through some processing, so they aren't the number one choice, but can be used in order to offer some variety to your meals.

- Wholegrain pasta, macaroni, spaghetti;
- High fiber (low sugar) whole grain breakfast cereals;
- Muesli;
- Grits;
- Oatcakes, rice cakes;
- Shredded Wheat;
- All Bran;
- Ryvita Crispbread;
- Corn Tortilla;
- Ezekiel Bread;
- Whole wheat pita or tortilla;
- Low carb flat bread.

Finally, another source of natural carbohydrate includes fruits such as:

- Apples, oranges, bananas, berries, pears, plums, peaches, melons, grapefruit, cranberries.

Fruits of course contain loads of nutrients, antioxidants and minerals which are great for our bodies. They are higher in sugar though, so during transformation periods they will be limited, and can be eaten more frequently during maintenance. It is best to have a higher intake of vegetables than fruits.

Carb sources such as whole grains, vegetables, fruits and beans promote good health by delivering vitamins, minerals and fiber to the body. Fiber is an important component to your diet. We need it to stay healthy. Fiber helps maintain our gastrointestinal tract cells and without enough of it, these cells can't stay healthy, your body will experience deficiencies, and toxins will be allowed to enter.

Fiber slows down the breakdown of starch and delays glucose absorption to the blood. It lowers cholesterol and helps control blood sugar levels, constipation, colon cancer, hemorrhoids, colitis and diverticulitis. You will feel more "full" when you eat foods that are higher in fiber because they take longer to chew. That "full" sensation lasts longer than if you eat foods that are low in fiber. Fiber is an important part of the equation when you are trying to lose weight so start reading labels and choose foods that are higher in fiber. A good source of fiber will have 2.5 grams or more per serving. If you currently have little fiber in your diet, please add it in slowly. If you add it too quickly, you may experience gastrointestinal discomfort in the form of gas, diarrhea and bloating.

Next, let's discuss timing of carbohydrates. Ideally, you will be eating four to seven times per day. The meals that should contain the highest amount of carbohydrates will be your first meal of the day and your post-workout meal. A breakfast high in carbohydrates is important because your body has been fasting all night while sleeping and needs to be refueled, and your metabolism needs to be jumpstarted for the day. Just like your mother told you, breakfast is in fact the most important meal of the day. If you skip breakfast, you are immediately sabotaging your fitness goals by putting your body into a muscle burning phase.

If you eliminate carbohydrates from your morning meal, you simply aren't going to be as efficient in your workouts or your daily life in general. Throughout the day, you should taper the amount of carbs you eat at each meal and avoid them (with the exception of vegetables) at your meals later in the day. The reason for this is that you are more active earlier in the day so your body will be able to utilize the energy from the carbs throughout the day. Later at night, as your metabolism begins to slow down, if you consume large amounts of carbs they won't be as easily used for energy. There is also a much higher likelihood that they will be stored in your body as fat.

Carbohydrates should always be consumed with a form of protein. You should never have a meal that is just carbs. Every meal should include protein.

Your body type can also be a factor in determining your carb intake. We will go over body types in a later chapter. If you have endomorphic tendencies (typically endomorphs gain fat weight easily), you may be more sensitive to carbohydrates and will thus be more successful on a program that supplies a lower amount of them.

In summary, carbohydrates are not your enemy. They are an essential part of your diet and are necessary for your body to function properly and to burn fat properly. What is most important is that you eat the right types of carbohydrates in the right portion sizes and at the right times of the day. The diet plans that are part of the Hitch Fit program are all based around these important key elements of carb consumption. Another part of what we do on the Hitch Fit online program is aid you in finding what a good carb intake level will be for you.

Fats

Fat. It's a dreaded word. Fats are a group of chemical substances in food that are generally insoluble (don't dissolve) in water. There are several classes. The most common are triglycerides, saturated, monounsaturated and polyunsaturated fats, cholesterol and phospholipids.

Although we have been conditioned to believe that all fats are bad for us, that simply is not the truth. In fact, we need fat in our diets on a daily basis in order to maintain good health and to function at our highest levels. Fats provide energy to the body but are calorically higher in density, so they are more likely to store as fat in your body if over-consumed. In the right portions and types, fats will actually benefit your health because they aid in cell function.

Just as with carbohydrates, the type of fats you consume, the time of day, and amount that you eat are the issues that must be addressed. All fats have nine calories per gram whereas carbohydrates and protein each have four calories per gram. Being calorically higher in density, it is important to consume them in little amounts throughout the day with most of your meals. The time to avoid including fats in your meals is pre- and post-workout. They have a much slower digestion rate, so if you consume them around workout times your body won't be able to digest and intake the protein and carbs it needs as efficiently as possible. Let's dive right into this final essential food category.

The Good Fats

Unsaturated fats are the ones that are so important for our bodies. They are the healthy fats that help us experience normal growth and development, store energy, provide cushioning for internal organs, maintain cell membranes, provide flavor, consistency and stability to our foods and help our bodies to absorb certain vitamins such as A, D, E, K and caretonoids. Healthy fats also help to lower our LDL cholesterol levels (which is the bad cholesterol that clogs up the arteries and can lead to numerous heart and health issues) and increase HDL levels (which is the "healthy" cholesterol). You want to have a high number of HDL. The good fats are a great source of energy for your body and will help you to avoid feeling lethargic.

There are two types of healthy fats: polyunsaturated and monounsaturated. Polyunsaturated fats have cholesterol-lowering properties. The most common types of polyunsaturated fats are Omega 3 and Omega 6. These are two essential fatty acids we must obtain from our diets because our bodies doesn't produce them. Most people take in more Omega 6 fatty acids, which come from plant sources, than Omega 3 fatty acids (which are also good for you and essential for health). Omega 3 fatty acids are found mostly in cold water fish, so if you aren't a big fish eater be sure that you are attaining your Omega 3 fatty acids in supplement form.

Monounsaturated fats are also good for your heart. They are the ones that help to lower the LDL cholesterol levels. Studies show that people who eat diets higher in monounsaturated fats typically live longer and have less incidence of developing cancer.

Here is a list of foods which should be used as your main source of good fats:

- Avocado;

- Olive oil, canola oil, peanut oil, grape seed oil, fish oil;

- Olives;

- Nuts (almonds, walnuts, peanuts, cashews, macadamia and most other nuts);

- Natural peanut butter, almond butter, cashew butter, macadamia nut butter;

- Corn, soybean, safflower and other cottonseed oils;

- Fish; and

- Flax seed, hemp seed.

The Bad Fats

The fats that you want to avoid are saturated fats, trans fats and hydrogenized fats. A lot of foods undergo a chemical process called hydrogenation during food processing in order to give them more flavor and a longer shelf life. It's best to limit the amount of these fats in your diet as much as possible especially when you are trying to lose weight. These fats will not only help you gain weight, they also increase LDL levels and are the main dietary cause of high cholesterol. Saturated fats are mostly derived from animal sources such as beef, beef fat, veal, lamb, pork, lard, poultry fat, butter, cream, milk, cheeses and other dairy products made from whole milk. They are also found in palm oil, coconut oil and palm kernel oil or cocoa butter.

When you are reading your ingredients labels, be sure to watch out for these. Trans fats (also known as partially hydrogenated fats) are found in a lot of unhealthy foods including: fried foods, crackers and cookies, any commercial snack product, vegetable oils and margarine. You should aim to keep these foods out of your diet completely. All they are going to do is hold you back from attaining your goals, and they are not good for your overall health.

The most important things to remember are that healthy fats are an essential part of your diet. Eat small portions of fats throughout the day. (Your Hitch Fit diet plan will show you the amounts and times that will be best for your body and goals.) Consume mostly unsaturated fats and essential fatty acids and limit how much cheese, red meat and butter you eat. Avoid fried foods and commercial snacks. You'll satisfy your body's cravings, protect yourself from heart disease, look better and feel stronger.

Liquids

When it comes to weight loss, you have to be aware of all calories that you are ingesting in a day. That includes liquid calories. It's amazing the hundreds and even thousands of calories per day that people are drinking, and are still trying to figure out why they aren't losing fat weight. Soda and fruit juices are basically sugar in a bottle. Because you don't fill up too quickly when you have a drink such as this, it is extremely easy to have your calorie intake go through the roof, even though you don't feel full.

These are all simple sugars, too, so they are very easily converted right into fat once you have consumed them. Sodas and fruit juices should be completely cut out of your diet. Some people will literally lose a couple of pounds right off the bat just by cutting out these sugary carbonated drinks. Diet sodas don't have the calories that regular soda has, but they can lead to weight gain by causing dehydration and a slow-down in your metabolism. In addition, they contain a lot of chemicals that will not allow your body to perform at optimum levels.

Another thing to be wary of is your morning caffeine kick. There's nothing wrong with a cup of coffee in the morning, but keep it straight coffee or espresso or tea. When you start getting fancy drinks with milk, whipped cream and caramel added to them, you would be amazed at how quickly the calories add up. Some of those drinks have almost 1,000 calories in them. For some people this is more than half of what they should be consuming in an entire day!

Alcohol is another liquid source of empty calories that leads to weight gain. Alcohol is a drug and is stored as fat in the body because it isn't a carbohydrate and can't be metabolized by your body unless it turns it into fat. It also causes protein deficiency and dehydration. It can stimulate your appetite too, so on top of drinking empty calories there is a good chance that you will consume excess calories!

Alcohol affects your reaction time, balance, and your eye/hand coordination. We are not saying that you have to eliminate alcohol from your lifestyle forever. Personally we don't drink because we choose to give 100% to our chosen path of life, and to be walking billboards for health and fitness. If you choose to include alcohol in your life, you must practice moderation and make good choices. Don't drink on a regular basis if you are serious about achieving your fitness goals, and especially if you are undergoing transformation. If you choose to drink, stay away from drinks that are sugary. (Margaritas, daiquiris and other fruity drinks are loaded with sugar.).

We've gone over what you shouldn't drink. What about what you should drink? The answer: water. Water is a vital element for your body to function properly. It is second only to oxygen.

You literally can't survive without water. 55 to 60% of your body weight is actually water weight. It aids in almost every basic function of your body including metabolism, temperature regulation, blood circulation and the ability of your body to flush out toxins and waste. Staying hydrated is critical to achieving your fitness goals. Having plenty of water in your body keeps your muscles full, speeds up your metabolism and helps you to feel full throughout the day. If you don't drink enough water, your body will actually start drawing water from the muscles themselves. Dehydration can cause fatigue and can even cause you to be moody.

Most people drink sodas and coffee and totally disregard drinking plain water. The minimum guidelines for water consumption say to drink six to eight glasses of water per day. In our opinion that is not enough. Especially since you are reading this book, indicating you are a Hitch Fit transformation in progress, or are soon to be a Hitch Fit transformation, which means you are going to be exercising regularly, sweating and needing to replenish that lost water. To figure out how much water you should be drinking, divide your body weight in pounds by two. You should be consuming a minimum of that amount in ounces of water per day.

**For example, if you weigh 200 pounds you should be consuming a minimum of 100 ounces of water in a day.

Drink water consistently throughout the day even if you don't actually feel thirsty. By the time your body actually tells you that you are thirsty you are already dehydrated. Another sign that you are dehydrated is the color of your urine. If you are drinking adequate amounts of water it should be a very light yellow color. If it is a dark yellow color, drink more water.

You need to drink just as much water in the winter time as in the summer time. Just because it isn't hot out and you aren't sweating as much doesn't mean that you don't have to drink as much. Your body needs water in order to stay warm just as much as it does to stay cool. I would advise you to keep a record of how much water you drink as you start your transformation process. You may be amazed at how little you are drinking!

Water is the single most important beverage you should be drinking on a consistent basis throughout the day.

You can still drink your coffee or tea (use sugar free sweeteners such as Splenda® and use skim milk instead of cream) but be sure that you are drinking enough water. If you think that water is too bland, you can use lemons, limes or cucumbers to add some flavor. You can also use sugar free drink mixes such as Crystal Lite®.

In conclusion, cut out the sodas and sugary drinks. Cut out or greatly moderate the amount of alcohol that you are consuming, especially during your transformation period. All of those unnecessary liquid calories are just going to hold you back from losing weight. Drink water, lots of water, every single day in order for your body to operate as efficiently as possible and in order to successfully lose weight.

Most Desirable Muscle Group

A set of six pack abs is hands down the most desired muscle group, and it is also probably the most challenging to attain. Sexy abs take HARD work, plenty of cardio and the number one, most important factor is consistently clean diet. It doesn't matter how many advertisements are on television saying you have to buy some silly gadget to get a six pack. It doesn't matter how convincing the infomercial models are at telling you they obtained their six packs in only 3 minutes of work a day. Honestly, you could work your abs all day every day and NEVER see them if your nutrition isn't on point and you are able to burn off the fat layers that are covering them up.

Crunches and core exercises are important for strengthening the abdominals, lower back and oblique muscles. They help you avoid back injuries, and core strength is important for controlling your upper and lower body. But the key to actually seeing the definition and visual effect of rippling abs is having a low percentage of body fat.

People write to us on a daily basis and want to know the secret of a shredded six pack and this is what we tell them: abs are all about your diet. That is the plain and simple truth. Everybody has a six pack set of abs, but if you don't reduce your body fat through sufficient cardio AND proper nutrition, you will never see them.

Food Labels and Ingredient Listings

Food labels can be very misleading. Don't be fooled into thinking a product is "healthy" or good for you because it says so on the label. Just because a label says "fat free" or "sugar free" doesn't mean that is necessarily true. Labeling laws are such that as long as a serving size contains less than a certain amount of fat, sugar or calories, it can be labeled as being "free" of that product.

For example a product can be labeled as "sugar free" if it contains less than ½ gram of sugar per serving. Another great example is "fat-free/ calorie-free" cooking sprays. If you read the label on the back of one of these cans you will see that a serving size is 1/3 second.

According to labeling laws, as long as a product has less than ½ gram of fat per serving it can be called "fat free," and if it has under 5 calories per serving, it can be called "calorie free." In a full second of spray, there are actually 7 calories. If there are 702 servings in a can (1/3 second) that means that there are 234 seconds of spray in a can which means in a "calorie free" product there are actually 1,638 calories. Cooking spray is of course a much better alternative than using butter or something heavily laden with calories, but just be aware that labels need to be looked at a little more closely and it's important to educate yourself on what the labels actually mean.

When checking out labels you should see what the carbohydrate content, fat content and protein content are per item. See how many sugars are in the product and also check out the serving size. I've seen a lot of "healthy" sports drinks that contain 2 ½ servings per bottle and have just as much sugar (if not more) as a bottle of soda. The same rule applies for a lot of supposedly healthy protein bars. Many of them are really high in sugar, and as you know, sugar converts to fat in your body. So, start reading the labels and if you choose to use protein bars as a supplement to your nutrition then choose the ones that are lower in sugar. A lot of these bars also contain unhealthy saturated fats and hydrogenated oils so it is a good idea to check out the ingredients list as well.

When reading an ingredient label, be aware that items are listed in the order of their prevalence. So if you pick up a product and the first ingredient is sugar or high fructose corn syrup, put it down and walk away. The same goes for products that contain trans fats and hydrogenated or partially hydrogenated products. If you are reading a label for a whole wheat product, the first ingredient should be whole wheat flour. If it says "enriched or bleached" it has undergone a process that has taken out most of the nutritional value.

Spicing up your foods

Don't be afraid to spice up your foods! Spices are a great, no calorie way to add variety too.

Common Diet Mistakes

Here are some common diet mistakes we strongly advise you to avoid because they will just hold you back from achieving your fitness goals.

1. Don't go on a crash diet...you know the ones I'm talking about, where all you eat is lettuce or jelly beans. You are starving your body and slowing down your metabolism, making it easier for your body to store fat. You are also losing precious lean muscle tissue.

2. Don't rely on the gym alone to achieve your fitness goals. The only way to completely transform your body is to properly nourish your body and live the right lifestyle by making positive healthy choices on a daily basis.

3. Don't think that you are being deprived. You have to keep a healthy mind set and a positive attitude about attaining your fitness goals. As soon as you start feeling bad for yourself because you can't have this cookie or that piece of cake the sooner you are going to cave to the cravings and temptation. If you realize that you are making the healthy and positive

choice to not have that type of food because your health, happiness and physical, mental, emotional and spiritual fitness are more important, you will not feel deprived. Instead, you will feel empowered at your ability to control your choices.

4. Don't think you can never enjoy your favorite treats again. Once you have achieved your fitness goals and your body is in a maintenance mode, you can enjoy your favorite foods in moderation. They can be incorporated into your fit and healthy lifestyle.

5. Don't forget that balance is the key to healthy nutrition. Stay away from overeating, or not eating enough which can be just as bad! Don't be afraid of carbohydrates and don't be afraid of fats. Just eat the right types in the right amounts.

6. Don't be a victim of cravings. Be prepared ahead of time. Know what you are going to eat and when you are going to eat it. Get yourself into a set eating schedule and have the foods that you need ready to go.

CHAPTER ELEVEN
FITNESS

There are five main components of fitness:

> ➤ Muscular endurance, which is the ability of a muscle to perform multiple repetitions of an exercise;

> ➤ Muscular strength, which is the maximum amount of force a muscle can exert;

> ➤ Cardiovascular endurance, which is the fitness level of the heart and lungs;

> ➤ Flexibility, which is the range of motion available at a given joint; and

> ➤ Body composition, which is the amount of lean body mass compared to fat mass.

All of these pieces of the fitness puzzle are equally important to obtain optimal fitness levels. You can work on improving all of these areas through strength training, cardiovascular training and stretching. A lot of people write to us and ask which one of these activities they should do to get in the best shape. The answer is "all of the above". In addition to eating properly, you need to do resistance training and cardio in order to optimize your fat loss results.

Strength Training

Strength training is important for everybody. If you want your body to have a toned and lean look, you must strength train. If you have never trained with weights, the idea may seem intimidating to you. Be assured that it is worth it, and it is essential to your success. You don't have to train at a big gym to sufficiently work your muscles. You can do this from the comfort and convenience of your own home in many instances.

If you enjoy working out in a gym setting, you can choose from all different types of facilities, including private studios where you work one on one with a trainer, women's only facilities, large corporate gyms, etc. It is important that you select a facility that feels right for you and commit to making that work out place your second home, especially during the course of your physical transformation.

Why should you strength train?

There are numerous benefits to training against resistance. You will build lean muscle mass, which by now we know leads to increased metabolism and faster fat burning capability. In fact, each pound of muscle you add increases your BMR (basal metabolic rate) by 3 to 5%. When you have increased muscle mass, your body has more room for stored fuel from your food sources. When the fuel (known as glycogen) stores in your muscles, it doesn't circulate through the blood to the liver where it is converted to fat. Rather it stores in the muscle and is available when you need the energy.

In addition to strengthening your muscles, you also strengthen your bones. This helps to prevent osteoporosis and bone density loss. You increase the stability of your ligaments and tendons, which will help to reduce the chances of injury at your joints. Strength training increases your functional capacity for completing everyday tasks or for enhanced performance while playing a sport. It also has mental and emotional benefits. It teaches discipline, raises your self-esteem and improves your self-confidence.

Strength training is hands down the most effective method of body shaping, strengthening and conditioning. Lean muscle takes up less space than fat. So as your body composition changes, you will lose inches and drop clothing sizes even if the scale doesn't show major differences in actual pounds lost. Strength training helps to improve posture and reduces your risk of lower back injury. When you strength train you are mainly working on increasing your muscular strength and endurance but you also make cardiovascular improvements when you train at higher intensity.

Strength Training Myths

There are some common misgivings about strength training, so we would like to address a few myths before going any further.

Myth #1 - Strength Training will make women bulky.

I hear this one over and over from women, "I don't want to use weights because I don't want to get big and bulky." Ladies, you aren't going to get big and bulky by strength training. When you see female bodybuilders or figure competitors who have more muscle mass, trust me, it didn't happen by accident. They have worked extremely hard in order to attain that level of muscularity.

Most women are going to have a difficult time building large muscles due to low levels of the testosterone hormone. No one is asking you to go in the gym and throw around huge weights. It's unnecessary and unless your goal is to become a bodybuilder and you start living, eating and training like a bodybuilder, your body simply isn't going to look like that. What you will develop are firm, strong and toned muscles that are aesthetically pleasing. You are going to decrease your body fat percentages and will have a smaller, tighter body that burns fat much more efficiently.

Myth #2 - You can lose fat from a specific area.

Not true. There is absolutely no such thing as "spot reduction." You can't say to your body, I want to lose weight in my thighs or around my belly. When you exercise you are using up energy and burning fat from all different parts of your body, not just one specific area, no matter how hard you work it.

The key to reducing the fat in your trouble spots is consistency and dedication to your program. Typically your body stores fat in the most stubborn areas first. For women this is the hips, thighs and buttocks. For men, this is around the abdomen. If it's the first place that you gain weight, it is probably one of the last places that you will lose weight. A woman who is a "pear" shape, with a larger bottom than top will probably start to lean out on her upper body first. Consistency with your diet, cardio and strength training program are the keys to eventually burning off the fat in those trouble spots. Those pills out now claiming to target fat in certain areas are bogus. That is just not true. It's absolutely not possible, so don't fall for the hype.

Myth #3 - The more you sweat, the more fat you lose.

Sweat is your body's cooling system. You will sweat more in hot weather and when you wear layered clothing than you will in cool weather. However, the weight that you are losing is just water weight and will come back as soon as you re-hydrate yourself. So, sitting in a steam room will not make you lose actual weight. Sweat can be a good indicator of how hard you are working out though. If you are working hard, sweating a lot is a good sign that you are burning a lot of calories and more fat.

Myth #4 - You can turn fat into muscle.

Fat and muscle are two totally different types of tissue and one doesn't convert into the other. When you stop exercising, your muscles will shrink and your metabolism will slow down, but the muscle tissue won't turn into fat. Vice versa, when you work out and are burning fat, the fat cells will shrink but they won't convert into muscle tissue.

Strength training programs should always include exercises for all the major muscle groups to ensure your body to be strong all around on the inside and out. You want your strength to be balanced in all parts of your body, front and back, side to side. You want your chest to be as strong as your back, your quadriceps to be as strong as your hamstrings, your biceps to be as strong as your triceps. It is important not to neglect certain muscle groups just because you don't enjoy training them as much. If your body is not balanced in its training you will have muscular imbalances. Muscular imbalances lead to one part of your body overcompensating for weakness in another part. This overcompensation puts added stress on your joints leading to postural deviations which over time lead to injury.

Body Type and Training

Some people seem to be able to lose weight or gain muscle much more quickly than others. Why is that? One big reason is that every single body is different and unique, so it is very important that you aspire to be the best YOU can be with what you have as opposed to trying to be exactly what someone else is. There are three main body types, and the type you are will influence how your body responds to training.

The first body type is the mesomorph. The mesomorph has an hourglass shape, typically broader at the shoulders and hips, narrower at the waist. This type of physique usually has a high muscle to fat ratio and a medium bone structure. People with a mesomorph physique can look fit even without exercise due to how symmetrical their bodies are. This body type will respond very well to strength training and to endurance training. They typically have a moderate metabolism and weight loss is a bit easier for them.

The second type is the endomorph. These bodies are round, soft and pear shaped with more fat distributed at the hips and thighs. Bone structure is medium to large and the muscles are not well defined. This body type has a higher fat to muscle ratio and shorter limbs relative to the trunk of the body. Their metabolism is slower so they need to work harder on endurance training in order to achieve weight loss. The endomorphs' diet may need to have a lower ratio of carbohydrates in it as they are typically more sensitive to carbohydrate insulin spikes and fat storage. Strength training usually comes easier for the endomorph.

The third type is the ectomorph. The ectomorph is going to be a "hard gainer," and putting on size and muscle is going to be more challenging for them. They have a high metabolism and will need to consume even more calories in order to maintain the muscle mass that is on their bodies. Physically, they have a long, rectangular shape, are flat-chested, with slender hips and no defined waist. In order to build muscle and grow, they will need to consume a higher percentage of carbohydrates. The ectomorph is poorly muscled and small boned with longer limbs as compared to the trunk of the body. The ectomorph can look like they have a low body fat percentage because they are typically thin due to the fast metabolism. But, in fact, unless they are strength training and eating properly, their fat-to-muscle ratio can be very high. A lot of ectomorphs are what is sometimes referred to as "skat" or skinny but fat. For example, a woman who is 120 pounds and appears small but has 30% body fat due to poorly developed muscle is at just as much risk of developing injury and health problems as someone who is visually overweight or obese.

You don't have to be all or nothing when it comes to body type. You may be a cross between two types. For example, you may be an endo-mesomorph where you have well-developed muscle but have a higher body fat level, which you tend to carry more in your hips or thighs.

You may be an endo-ectomorph, meaning you are small boned, long limbed and poorly muscled with a layer of fat that is typically carried in the hips and thighs.

Or perhaps you are an ecto-mesomorph, meaning you have well-defined muscles but you are still long, thin and wiry.

Regardless of what body type you are, you can transform your physique into the best it can be through exercise and proper nutrition. Knowing your body type will just make it easier to determine what type of training is best for you.

How to Strength Train

How should you strength train? Strength training programs should include exercises for all of the major muscle groups (please refer to the Hitch Fit DVD and the Hitch Fit online website for more specific information on exercises to do and proper form). What should your intensity levels be and how frequently should you train? There isn't a cookie cutter answer for this one. If you are just starting out and are new to the strength training scene you may only be strength training two to three days per week. If you are an experienced, intermediate or advanced exerciser you may be strength training four to six days per week. The duration of your training sessions will vary, also.

There is no set amount of time that you have to be in the gym. You can get a killer workout in 20 minutes and be more efficient than someone who is dawdling around the gym for two hours.

There are so many different styles of strength training out there, and we are not going to say that any of them are wrong, but we believe we have developed a highly effective style of training that will get you real, long-lasting results. The programs we are going to provide you through Hitch Fit are based on a style we have developed over the years. We have seen countless people transform their bodies, including online clients and in-person clients, based on these training techniques.

Our training style focuses on keeping the intensity high for clients interested in losing weight and burning body fat, or for sport-specific athletes. If this describes you, regardless of what fitness level you currently have, the goal is to push yourself to your greatest potential during each workout.

If you are a beginner, you need to increase your cardiovascular and muscular endurance at the same time as your strength endurance, so our workouts will include a variety of cardio movements intertwined with resistance training exercises. The goal of the workouts is to burn as many calories as possible and to work your muscles to fatigue and even to failure.

These workouts are efficient with little rest time. Long periods of rest are not beneficial when your goal is to burn body fat and get a lean, toned or chiseled physique. There is no need to be lifting heavy weights and then taking two minutes of rest time.

When I train clients in person, their workouts are never the same. It is a new program each and every time they step into the gym. The focus is not on counting repetitions and tracking a certain amount of weight they can lift. It's about burning out those muscles and challenging the body as much as we can.

You must challenge your body to change it. Hitch Fit provides workouts that will do just that. Ultimately the goal of this program is for you to learn enough about your own body and how it responds to strength training that you can effectively train yourself for the rest of your life.

Just as critical as selecting the right workout routine is making sure you switch up that routine at least every four weeks. You've probably heard of people with a lot of weight to lose dropping a bunch of weight when they initially start a new training program, and then suddenly their body stops changing. The reason is because they are no longer shocking their body, and it has reached what is known as a plateau. Their body has basically become so efficient at doing their workouts that it takes less energy expenditure and less calorie burning to get the job done.

Think of it this way. You start a new job and are unfamiliar with your new office, your new computer, your new co-workers, the lay out, the proper protocol for completing tasks. For your first couple of weeks it may take you a lot longer to complete simple tasks because you are in the learning phases of properly doing everything.

Within a couple of months, though, you have the system down and you are extremely efficient at what you do, so tasks that used to take an hour to complete can be done in 10 minutes. You don't need to use as much energy as you did when you first started because you are efficient. The same thing happens in your body. It adapts to a certain training program, becomes very efficient at doing it and then can go on autopilot to complete it. Therefore, you must challenge yourself and switch things up on a regular basis in the gym in order to avoid plateaus.

Types of Training

Here are some great techniques you can incorporate into your strength training programs that will allow you to continually shock your body.

- Giant Set - Moving rapidly from one exercise to the next for a series of 6-7 or more movements with little rest in between.

- Tempo or Slow Training - Performing a movement very slowly. For example, a three count up and a three count down. Keep it at this pace through the entire set.

- Pause Reps - Pausing part way through an exercise and holding the contraction for 2-3 seconds or more before continuing with the full repetition.

- Speed Training - Performing movements at a higher pace with lower weights.

- Isometric Training - Keeping a muscle contraction without actually moving your joint through a range of motion. This is what we want you to do all the time with your abs. Keep them tight and hold an isometric contraction regardless of what exercise you are doing.

- Superset - A series of two to three exercises performed back to back without resting. This can be different muscle groups or the same muscle group.

- Drop Set - Doing one exercise for a specific number of sets and repetitions per set. There is no rest between sets, and the amount of weight is dropped each set.

- Negative Training - Maintaining tension in your muscles and moving slowly and controlled through the portion of the exercise that would typically be the relaxation phase.

⬩ Plyometrics - These are high-intensity movements, such as high knees, burpees or jumping jacks, which you should only be able to perform for short periods of time.

You will find demonstrations of the different training styles and plyometric movements in your Hitch Fit DVD.

The Mind/Muscle Connection

The mind/muscle connection is an extremely important concept to incorporate into your training program. Basically this means that you develop a connection between the muscle group that is working and your mind. We've seen people in the gym swinging weights around with no awareness of what their body is actually doing. When you utilize the mind/muscle connection, essentially you are training "on purpose" rather than just letting your body mindlessly go through movements.

Eventually you may feel a burn or experience muscle fatigue, but if you actually focus on your muscles and pay attention to what they are doing and how they are doing it, you can fatigue them much more quickly and train them much more effectively. When you are working a particular muscle group, think about exactly what it is doing. Contract or tighten the muscle and keep it tight, regardless of whether you are in the contraction phase (the hard part of the exercise when you are tightening your muscle) or the down phase (or the relaxation phase).

Using the biceps curl as an example, before you even begin the curling movement upward tighten your biceps, keep it tight as you curl the weight up and in and then hold that contraction in your biceps throughout the entire movement. Don't let that muscle relax until your set is completely finished.

The same concept can be applied when you are doing your cardio. Be engaged with what you are doing, pay attention to your body, contract your muscles and put more force into what you are doing. Avoid zoning out and reading a book or watching television. You can burn far more calories by training on purpose and using your mind to attain the full capacity of your muscles.

Additional Tips for Strength Training

You should always warm up prior to strength training. A warm up can be three to five minutes of a light cardio activity. Basically the point is to get your body prepared for exercise by elevating the heart rate and warming up the muscles and joints so that they are ready to work.

Maintain proper posture when you are strength training. You will be able to work your muscles most effectively when your body is in proper alignment. Your feet should be parallel and shoulder- to hip-width apart, your knees should be slightly bent and not locked out, and your hips should be in a neutral alignment (not arching your back). In order to do this, keep the abdominal and lower pelvic muscles tight at all times.

Shoulders should be back and pressed down and in line with your hips. Your head should be in neutral alignment with your spine, and your ears should be in alignment with your shoulders.

Proper form is crucial when you are performing your movements. Don't compromise your form in order to lift heavier weights. When your form is not proper, you are usually not effectively working the muscle group you are trying to target. For proper form demonstrations of each exercise, please review the Hitch Fit DVD and log on to the online community (www.HitchFit.com) for additional video and guidelines.

You must be sure that you are always breathing throughout your exercises. Your body needs oxygen in order to exercise. It may sound silly, but in fact a lot of people have a tendency to hold their breath while they are strength training. Be sure you are taking deep inhales and exhales during every movement. Be especially aware of this if you have high blood pressure because if you hold your breath during exercise your blood pressure will rise.

Typically, you will inhale on the relaxation or easier part of an exercise, and exhale on the contraction phase or the hard part where you are actually pushing, pulling or lifting the weight. For example, when performing a push up you would inhale on the downward movement towards the floor and exhale as you push up and contract your chest, triceps and shoulder muscles.

Sleep

Sufficient sleep is essential to achieving your fitness goals. During sleep, your body is going through an important recovery cycle. When you work out, you are breaking down your muscles. The time when you actually gain strength is during your recovery periods when your body is rebuilding and repairing. If you get adequate amounts of sleep, your body will be able to repair properly, and you will be stronger for your next work out.

Adequate rest is just as important as adequate time spent in the gym. If you have a muscle group that is still extremely sore, that means it has not recovered properly yet. You should avoid working that muscle group directly and give it time to rebuild. If you keep working out without enough sleep and recovery time, you will continue to break down your muscles. They won't even have a chance at building and getting stronger.

Additionally, not getting enough sleep can hinder fat loss. The reason is because when you don't sleep, your body increases it's levels of the fat storing hormone known as cortisol. When cortisol levels are higher, your body will easily and readily store food as fat and it will fight against allowing your body to release fat as fuel. Getting enough sleep is a crucial piece of the fat loss puzzle.

There are four stages of sleep. The third and fourth stages are the most important for muscle recovery because this is when the brain enters REM (Rapid Eye Movement), so called because the eyes move back and forth under the lids. During REM sleep the brain resets chemicals in the emotional centers and clears short term memory banks. Without enough REM sleep, people become cranky and depressed, their memory and judgment are impaired, and they perform poorly on tests and reaction time. Sleep deprivation causes the body to lose the hormone leptin, which tells the body when it should feel full. When leptin drops the body starts to crave carbs. With low levels of leptin, your body will crave carbohydrates, even if you have had enough calories.

Some sure signs you aren't getting enough rest are if you have trouble waking up in the morning, are tired and cranky throughout the day, always need to have the alarm clock go off in order to wake up, doze off while watching television at night, rely on caffeine to stay awake throughout the day, frequently wake up during the night or take an exceptionally long time to recover from muscle soreness and fatigue. In addition to preventing your body from recovering from workouts, lack of sleep also affects your ability to concentrate and focus and weakens your immune system.

Sleep is critical for your physical, emotional and mental energy levels. Adults should get about seven hours of sleep per night. If you are working out hard, it is actually a good idea to take a nap in the afternoon. A 20- to 30- minute nap can revitalize you and again aid in muscle recovery. Catching these extra Z's in the afternoon is equivalent to an extra two hours of sleep.

Avoid drinking caffeine at least a few hours before going to bed, and if you have trouble sleeping, a warm shower before bed can help. When you are getting enough sleep at night, you won't even need an alarm clock to wake up, and it is a good idea to wake up at the same time each day, regardless of whether you need to, so that your body is on an efficient time table.

Cardio

Cardiovascular or aerobic exercise is any activity that uses large muscle groups in a continuous, rhythmic fashion for a sustained period of time. Cardio is necessary to keep you heart and lungs healthy and to burn enough calories to lose body fat. There are all different types of cardio activities that you can perform. Some of the most popular are running or jogging, walking, swimming, cycling, jumping rope, dancing, step aerobics, rowing or elliptical machine.

The amount of cardio you need if your goal is to burn body fat and lose weight varies from person to person and depends on a number of factors. These include how many calories you consume, the intensity level of your workouts, your metabolism, age and gender, your body fat percentage and weight, and your exercise schedule.

For cardio to be as effective as possible, your calorie expenditure needs to exceed your calorie consumption. One pound of fat is 3,500 calories, so in order to burn a pound of fat in a week you need to expend 3,500 calories more than you are consuming throughout the course of a week. The amount of time you spend doing your cardio isn't as important as the amount of calories you are expending during your session.

We typically advise clients to track the calories they are burning as opposed to doing a set number of minutes. To be sure you are burning enough calories, set a number goal for yourself at the beginning of the week and make sure that you hit this number or exceed it by weeks' end. If your goal is to expend 3,500 calories, then you can break that number up however you would like. If you want it over the course of seven days, that means you have to burn 500 calories per day in cardio. If you want to complete this number in five days, that means you have to burn 700 calories per day to hit it.

Let's say in 60 minutes you burned 600 calories. That's 10 calories per minute, which is a moderate intensity level. The higher intensity level at which you exercise, the more quickly you are going to burn calories. Eventually you want to work up to 15 to 20 calories per minute in order to burn 1,000 to 1,200 total calories in that hour. If you aren't doing your cardio on a machine and you need to get an estimate of how many calories you have expended, calculate 10 to 15 calories per minute depending on how intensely you were working out.

To get the most from your workouts, work within your target heart rate, which is what challenges your cardio-respiratory system and enables you to put your body in the training or aerobic zone. Within this zone, your body burns a higher percentage of fat calories; therefore, it is commonly referred to as the fat-burning zone.

This is how we will calculate your target heart rate:

Heart-rate reserve = maximal heart-rate - resting heart-rate.

Maximal heart rate is the highest rate a person can attain during exercise. While an electrocardiogram test would provide the most accurate MHR, for practical application an age-predicted heart-rate formula was developed.

Maximal heart-rate = 220 – age.

This formula is based on the assumption that one's heart rate at birth is 220 and decreases by one every year. The accuracy of determining maximal heart-rate based on this formula can vary at any given age by + 10 beats per minute.

Resting heart rate is the rate at which your heart beats at full rest. To determine your resting heart rate, take your pulse before getting out of bed, counting the pulse for a full 60 seconds, three mornings in a row and average the counts.

As your cardiovascular endurance improves, you will be able to work at higher intensity levels, and your heart rate will not elevate as quickly. The lower your heart rate stays when you are working at higher intensities, the better shape your heart and lungs are in. Your recovery heart rate is also a good indicator of cardiovascular fitness. The more quickly your heart rate drops back down to normal after being elevated during a workout, the better condition your heart is in.

Your metabolism is another factor to consider when determining how much cardio you need. The higher your metabolism is, the less cardio you will have to do. The slower your metabolism is, the more cardio you will need. Factors such as age, gender, body fat and weight all affect how fast your metabolism is going to be. Metabolism is usually higher the younger you are, and men often have a higher metabolic rate than women. The higher your body fat percentage is, the slower your metabolism will be.

If you set a cardio goal for yourself in a given week, ate the proper amount of calories, hit your calorie expenditure goal and didn't lose weight, you need to increase the amount of cardio that you are doing. Unless you have a metabolic disorder or thyroid dysfunction, the problem is that you didn't expend more calories than you consumed.

In my opinion, the best time for cardio for those of you interested in burning body fat and losing weight is when you wake up in the morning before your first meal. Your body has been in a fasting state for six to nine hours while sleeping and by doing your cardio early in the morning your body must use fat storage as your source of energy.

Eat your first meal of the day, a good combination of carbs and protein, within 30 minutes or so of finishing your morning cardio. If you must have something in your stomach pre-cardio, have a shake with one to two scoops of whey protein powder. If morning cardio is simply not an option, then do it either in the afternoon, on a lunch break or after your strength training workout.

Research has shown that higher intensity cardio is more beneficial for fat-burning purposes than long slow cardio workouts, so keep those intensity levels up.

A Special Note for Hard Gainers

Now, let's take a moment and talk about the unique training style that is necessary for those of you who are hard gainers. As we've already covered, a hard gainer is naturally skinny. No matter what he or she eats, they seem to maintain the same body weight. Micah is a hard gainer, so adding muscle to his frame has taken a great deal of effort over a long period of time.

The training style for a hard gainer is going to be three to five days per week of resistance training with very light cardio. Sprinting or light walking one to two days per week are going to be the best forms of cardio for a hard gainer to reduce body fat without burning up precious muscle mass. Exercises should be performed using slow and controlled movements with longer rest periods, repetitions are going to be lower, and weight will be increased over time so that you are progressively getting stronger and gaining muscle mass. Workouts will to be 45 to 60 minutes long.

Basically you want to limit your caloric expenditure so that you aren't losing muscle. If you are trying to add mass onto your body, you need to be consuming more calories than you are expending. In some instances, this can be up to 24 times the number of pounds you weigh.

Flexibility

Stretching and flexibility are important components to your training regimen. Stretching should be done when your body is warmed up. Avoid stretching when your muscles are cold because you could easily pull or tear something. Think of your muscles as a piece of taffy. When warm, it stretches easily, but when cold, it will snap and break. Stretching is important because it helps restore and maintain a full range of motion at the joints. It keeps the joints lubricated so they can move properly. It helps to relax the body and mind and reduces muscle soreness. It allows for improved neuromuscular coordination and decreases your risk of injury. It also enhances balance and improves posture.

You can and should stretch every day. Stretches should be performed in a slow and controlled manner. You should hold each stretch for at least 15 to 20 seconds or longer. When you are stretching, remember to breathe, and each time you exhale, relax a bit deeper into your stretch. Don't move beyond your comfort zone while stretching. You should feel tension in your muscles and slight discomfort but not outright pain.

Typically you want to perform static stretches, meaning you move into your stretch and hold it. Avoid bouncing and jerking movements as those will increase your risk of pulling a muscle. Please review the Hitch Fit DVD for stretching demonstrations.

Tips for eating out or on the go

The more consistent you are with your nutrition the more quickly you are going to achieve results. Because we live busy lives you will probably be eating some meals out or on the go. Here are some tips on how to stick with your nutrition plan even in these situations.

1. It is better to eat than not eat. Don't starve yourself and go for longer than 2-3 hours without eating. Even if you are stuck with less than ideal nutritional sources please feed your body something to avoid losing muscle.

2. Be prepared. It is essential that you set aside time to have the foods that you need prepared in advance. Set aside time in the evening or get up a bit earlier in the morning to prepare your foods for the day. Shakes that you will need for the day can be prepped the night before and stored in the refrigerator. Take time on weekends to cook larger quantities of the foods that you will eat most frequently including turkey, chicken, sweet potatoes or brown rice. Store extra in the fridge or freezer. Fish is not going to last as long, so that should be prepared fresh.

3. Here are some items that will help you with your food prep. Keep them easily accessible (and USE them!): Digital food scale; measuring cups; tablespoons and teaspoons; blender; Tupperware to pack your mini meals in; and a cooler to carry your foods with you throughout the day.

4. When eating out, order items such as grilled chicken or fish. Never

be afraid to modify your meal selections. Even if grilled chicken isn't on the menu, ask your server for it. Most restaurants have chicken and will prepare it how you want if you ask. Always ask for no sauces, butters, oils or dressings to be put on your chicken or fish. Be specific about this because restaurants love to slather on all kinds of stuff for taste. You don't want those unnecessary calories because a lot of them are fat! When eating at a restaurant always get a protein source. If you are eating a meal where you are supposed to have a carb source (like breakfast), just be careful with how much you eat. If you are out to dinner with friends, skip the carb source (potato, rice etc…) and just ask for extra vegetables. Regardless of what a menu says, ask for what you want. If you ask politely, you will usually get what you need.

The hardest places to eat clean are going to be Italian (which is mostly pasta dishes) or Mexican (although you can usually get chicken and veggies). The best places are going to be sandwich or salad shops, or seafood/steak houses. Outback steakhouse is EXCELLENT at modifying the foods that you need. Order your chicken or fish with veggies (broccoli, asparagus or spinach are going to be your best choices). Specify that you want them steamed and nothing added to them!

5. Stay away from creamy dressings completely. Order dressings on the side and stick with a vinaigrette or low fat or no fat alternative and only use it for dipping. That is if you must have a dressing! You can also use things like lemon juice, pepper, vinegar or even Splenda® on your salads. When ordering house salads, find out what is on them. Ask to have them without cheese, bacon, croutons etc.

6. If you are eating at a friends' house, don't be afraid to ask them what they are having to eat. Offer to bring something and bring along food that you can eat. There are going to be people along the way who think the way that you are eating is crazy, but that's ok. If you are serious about achieving your fitness goals, you have to be serious about how you eat day in and day out.

If you over do it when you eat out, don't freak out. Just get back on your normal nutrition plan. If you need to cheat on your diet, only have one cheat meal, and limit it to once per week. Don't do a cheat day as this could set you back and eliminate an entire weeks' worth of progress. Cheat with types of foods as opposed to binging on a ton of extra calories.

Are you ready to step on stage?

Perhaps you have read this book and you are at a different stage of the game. Instead of just wanting to lose weight for health reasons, your goal is to step foot on stage and compete! Maybe your goal is to be a bikini model, a male or female fitness model or a figure athlete. If that is the case, then good for you! It is an awesome and amazing challenge to take on. It takes a level of drive and discipline that the majority of the population, do not possess. Seeing a competition prep through, and stepping on stage, can be one of the most empowering experiences you will ever go through.

Your nutrition will be strict. If you want to be successful, your focus will have to be on you. You could possibly lose some friends on the way who don't think that you're "fun" any more. To be honest, you have to be self-focused to train for a show. If you're not then you won't be giving yourself your best chance at success.

The most important thing as you enter the world of competition is to keep in mind that it is a subjective sport. Now you never know, you may be the next big thing. You may end up gracing the covers of multiple magazines, and you may, down the line, be one of the top names in the fitness industry. You'll never know until you take those first steps. But remember, even if you don't take first place in your shows, that doesn't mean that you aren't amazing.

The journey to the stage is about so much more than winning. It's about seeing what you're made of, and it's about overcoming all the obstacles and excuses that you may have let stand in your way. It's about seeing what the best YOU is. Don't dwell on comparing yourself to others. You have special gifts that no one else possesses, and your story is unique to you. No matter if you step on stage at a small local show in your hometown, or if you step on stage at the biggest world championships competition with the top names in the industry, YOUR story is going to inspire someone. It may be a family member, people who see your dedication and discipline at the gym, or someone who reads about your story in a magazine or on a website, or who sees your before pictures and can relate to your exact body type.

The worst thing you can do is not try. If it's in your heart to compete, then go for it. You'll never know how far you can go if you don't put yourself out there and try. There are people out there who think that if you aren't genetically blessed that you shouldn't step on stage. We disagree! If it's a challenge that you want to undertake, then don't procrastinate. See what you're made of and see what you can become. Some of the most amazing and inspiring transformation stories are from people who may not have the genetics to be at the top of the game, but overcame the most obstacles to get to be their personal best.

The training is hard and the nutrition is strict, there's no doubt about that. You will be tired, you will have cranky days, you will have moments where you want to break down and cry, but keep going, keep pushing and get to the goal. It's worth it.

CHAPTER TWELVE
FINAL THOUGHTS

Hitch Fit is constantly growing and thriving. By the time this book is published, we hope to have even more ways to reach out to our clients to add more value to this program through support, information and inspiration. We encourage you to communicate with us. We are very active on the social networks so please find us on Facebook and Twitter, and continue to watch the Hitch Fit website: www.HitchFit.com to see new additions there.

We will constantly be adding:

- ❖ New information;

- ❖ New workouts and ideas; and

- ❖ New fitness and nutrition information.

We invite and encourage your participation and feedback in our ever growing community!

The main purpose of this book is to provide additional information and education for our current clients. We also know that there are many of you reading this book who are curious about Hitch Fit that we haven't yet had the opportunity to work with. Regardless of which category you fall in, we truly hope that you enjoyed this book, and were able to glean useful information that will aid you in achieving your own personal transformation.

Your key to success is to take this program seriously. Every component is crucial to your success. You must train hard, eat right and push yourself as though we were standing there watching over your shoulder and telling you to keep on going. We are not mean trainers and we aren't too keen on yelling, but we do have big expectations of you because we know you are capable! Whether we are meeting in person or working together online, we are not tolerant of excuses because we know that when your health, fitness and ultimate transformation are a top priority in your life, you will find a way to succeed and achieve your goals. Keep striving to do the best you can do and be the best you can be. Always remember we are here for you. We are a team. We consider your success to be our success!

We hope that you can sense how sincere we are about wanting to share the best information with you that we possibly can. From the bottom of our hearts we want you to succeed. We know how good you are going to feel when you DO succeed. We are honored and thrilled to be a part of this journey with you!

- Micah and Diana -

Website resources:

Hitch Fit: www.HitchFit.com

Hitch Fit Gym: www.HitchFitGym.com

Diana's personal site: www.DianaChaloux.com

Micah's personal site: www.MicahLacerte.net

Twitter: http://www.Twitter.com/HitchFit

http://www.twitter.com/DianaChaloux

Twitter Hitch Fit Hashtag Community

#RUHitchFit #IAMHitchFit

**Use these hashtags in your Twitter posts to join in the Hitch Fit conversations with online and in person clients worldwide. Tweet about your workouts, your healthy nutrition choices, overcoming obstacles, anything that has to do with your Hitch Fit lifestyle!

Diana and Micah on YouTube:

Diana's Channel: Behind the scenes at competitions, workouts, photo shoots, and fun silly clips from life!

http://www.YouTube.com/shoobydoo52

Micah's Channel: Great workout tips, competition footage, and more fun footage from Micah and Diana's lives!

http://www.YouTube.com/MMLacerte

MySpace:

Diana's: http://www.MySpace.com/fitdiana

Micah's: http://www.MySpace.com/MicahLacerte

Facebook:

http://www.FaceBook.com/HitchFit

Made in the USA
Lexington, KY
18 June 2012

	Item Price	Total
	$12.99	$12.99

	$12.99
ng	$1.59
	$1.38
	$15.96
it	$15.96
	$0.00

ng.

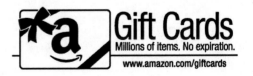

amazon.com

DSZN   SP

Your order of June 18, 2012 (Order ID 105-3085066-7207409)

Qty.	Item
1	**Hitch Fit: Keys to Transforming Your Life** Paperback (** P-1-Q36F123 **) 145286523X

Subtotal
Shipping & Han
Tax Collected
Order Total
Paid via credit/
Balance due

This shipment completes your order.

Have feedback on how we packaged your order? Tell us at www.amazon.com/packa